BRENT Q. HAFEN is Professor of Health Sciences at Brigham Young University. He is the author of sixteen books in the field of food, nutrition, alcohol and drug abuse, and related health topics.

PRENTICE-HALL INTERNATIONAL, INC., *London*
PRENTICE-HALL OF AUSTRALIA PTY. LIMITED, *Sydney*
PRENTICE-HALL OF CANADA, LTD., *Toronto*
PRENTICE-HALL OF INDIA PRIVATE LIMITED, *New Delhi*
PRENTICE-HALL OF JAPAN, INC., *Tokyo*
PRENTICE-HALL OF SOUTHEAST ASIA PTE. LTD., *Singapore*
WHITEHALL BOOKS LIMITED, *Wellington, New Zealand*

HOW TO LIVE LONGER

BRENT Q. HAFEN
with Kathryn J. Frandsen

A SPECTRUM BOOK

PRENTICE-HALL, INC., Englewood Cliffs, New Jersey 07632

Library of Congress Cataloging in Publication Data

HAFEN, BRENT Q.
   How to live longer.

   (A Spectrum Book)
   Includes bibliographical references and index.
   1. Health.   2. Longevity.   3. Diseases—Causes and
theories of causation.   I. Title.
RA776.H134   613   81-2142
ISBN 0-13-415265-4   AACR2
ISBN 0-13-415257-3 (pbk.)

© 1981 by Prentice-Hall, Inc., Englewood Cliffs, New Jersey 07632

A SPECTRUM BOOK

10   9   8   7   6   5   4   3   2   1

Printed in the United States of America

Editorial/production supervision and interior design by Frank Moorman
Cover design by Velthaus & King
Manufacturing buyer: Barbara A. Frick

CONTENTS

CHRONIC
AND COMMUNICABLE DISEASES, 104

CONSUMER HEALTH, 152

INDEX, 191

HOW TO LIVE LONGER

INTRODUCTION

How long will you live?

The answer depends on you—on how much you eat, on where you live, on whether you sleep with a window open, on whether you eat fresh fruits and vegetables (an apple a day?), on whether you wear a seat belt, on whether your grandfather had a stroke, on how many times you climb the stairs to your dorm room, on how much you earn during your lifetime, on how many cigarettes you smoke every day. All of those factors—and many more—determine not only how long you will live but what kind of life you will live.

And the important thing is that *you* have control over most of those factors. Of course, none of us can control whether our grandmother suffered a heart attack at the age of sixty or whether our father died from cancer of the colon. But each of us does control many other things that decide how soon we will die and how healthy we will be until then.

Not too many years ago medicine was a mystery. People didn't think about sickness (or wellness, for that matter) until they came down with a rumbling stomach, a stabbing earache, a throbbing head. First there was the trip to the bathroom medicine cabinet: There, in the bleary light, they fumbled along the crowded shelves, fingering first one bottle and then another, holding each up to squinting eyes, struggling to read the fading lines of ancient prescriptions. Finding just the remedy, they'd pop off the plastic lid, nestle a few brightly colored capsules in the valley of their tongue, and wash the remedy down with a few swigs of lukewarm water from the mug that sits on the edge of the sink.

Sometimes symptoms went away after a few trips to the medicine chest and a few resurrections of remedies past. Other times the symptoms persisted; some even got worse. The phone book was pulled out of the top drawer. A finger

1

followed the columns on a dogeared page to the scribbled-in number of the family doctor; an appointment was made for the day after tomorrow.

The doctor's waiting room was paneled in dark wood; tattered magazines —*Popular Mechanics, Parents, Good Housekeeping*—were scattered across end tables and empty vinyl-cushioned chairs. An elderly man settled in the corner, nodding sleepily. A mother cuddled a feverish baby in a woolen afghan; a teenager with his ankle bound in adhesive tape fidgeted nervously with the edge of his shirt. A middle-aged woman occupied the end seat; a rasping cough shook her entire body as she held a stained cotton handkerchief up to her mouth.

One by one they entered the inner sanctum, where a pleasant nurse weighed them, measured their blood pressure, jabbed a thermometer under their tongue. One by one they were led to small, humid examining rooms with multicolored slatted blinds at the windows. They gingerly took off their clothes—all of them—and folded them neatly in a pile in the corner on a cold metal stool, and they clutched firmly at the white sheet draped over them for modesty.

After a few minutes—long enough to read another article or two in one of the well-fingered magazines—in came the doctor, a brown rubber stethoscope hanging around his or her neck and a clipboard in hand. There were questions: How long has this pain bothered you? Have you been coughing? Do you notice a ringing in your ears when you bend over like this? Are your periods regular? Has anyone in your family ever had diabetes? Do you feel lonely often?

The doctor set the clipboard (now decorated with the answers to the seemingly disjointed questions) on the cluttered countertop and peered suspiciously under first one corner of the sheet, then another. There were grunts, biting of the lip, and a few well-placed pokes. The doctor scrawled out a prescription on a small square pad, tore off the top sheet, set it on the counter, hung the clipboard on a nail near the door, and disappeared down the hallway to the next examining room.

They carried the prescription to a drugstore on the corner of a busy street, where a stern pharmacist peered over the counter, hunched over bottles full of potions, and handed a small bottle and its taped-on label over the counter. Unsure of what they had—or why, or what caused them to be sick in the first place, or whether they could have prevented it—tens of thousands of Americans each year balanced those small prescription bottles on nightstands or counters next to the kitchen sink, and swallowed millions of capsules and tablets in hope of a cure.

All that has changed now.

We still go to the doctor; today's team of medical scientists is armed with information and techniques undreamed of by doctors even one or two decades ago. We still get prescriptions for medication, and we still pay for the bottles of potions and pills. Some of us still even try to treat ourselves with the bounties of the bathroom medicine chest.

But we have control now. We know more about our bodies, and we are learning more now than we have ever known before. We know more about how

Introduction

to choose a doctor; we can discuss intelligently the results of lab tests, the therapeutic value of various kinds of treatments. We can participate in our own health care because we know more about disease and what causes it. We know how drugs act on our bodies and what benefits and side effects we can expect from them. If you don't know as much about any of these things as you should, this book will help you learn.

And, most importantly, we know how to *prevent* disease. We have discovered what causes disease; we know what risk factors are involved. And we know how to reduce our risk of developing disease—even such serious diseases as cancer, heart disease, and emphysema—and how to increase our chances of living a long, healthy, happy life.

You are lucky because you live in an age when you are able to reap the benefits of years of medical research. Scientists and technologists have worked for years across the United States in sterile laboratories and overcrowded hospitals, spending billions of dollars to complete extensive research in the field of medicine.

How does that research benefit you?

We know now what factors contribute to longevity—and, as a result, what factors contribute to disease. We have identified the leading health problems in the United States. And we know what the leading causes of death are in the United States. Most of them are diseases, but we know what factors contribute to those diseases, and we know who runs a greater risk of developing those diseases. That means *you* can determine whether you are at risk—you can know whether you stand a greater than average chance of falling prey to one of those top ten killers, and you can take the steps you need to to remove yourself from that risk situation.

THE STATE OF THE UNION

The health of the American people has never been better; as Americans, we are healthier today than we have ever been.[1] Our ability to treat and prevent disease has grown tremendously through our understanding of what causes disease. A report released by the Surgeon General's Office at the beginning of the 1980's indicated that increased medical care and greater health expenditures have brought about an improved state of health—but that disease prevention and the promotion of health are even greater factors in the improvement. President Jimmy Carter, in an introduction to the report, stated:

We have come to take the seemingly miraculous cures of modern medicine almost for granted. And we tend to forget that our improved health has

3

come more from preventing disease than from treating it once it strikes. Our fascination with the more glamorous "pound of cure" has tended to dazzle us into ignoring the often more effective "ounce of prevention." I have long advocated a greater emphasis on preventing illness and injury by reducing environmental and occupational hazards and by urging people to choose to lead healthier lives.[2]

We can do better. In a period of two decades—from 1960 to 1978—the amount of money we as a nation spent on health care increased more than 700 percent, yet the increase has not yielded the striking improvements we might have hoped for. Why? Most of the money has been aimed at treatment and rehabilitation rather than prevention.[3]

Some strides in prevention have been gained, but we still lag behind a number of industrial nations. Twelve others do better in preventing deaths from cancer; twenty-six others have a lower death rate from circulatory disease. Eleven others do a better job of keeping babies alive during the first year of life. Fourteen others have a higher level of life expectancy for men, and six others have a higher level for women.[4]

We can do better—we can begin to approach our potential—if we realign our priorities, if we make a solid commitment to develop better health habits, and if we identify and assess risks on an individual basis in order to prevent the initial occurrence of disease.

CONTRIBUTORS TO HEALTH

A number of overlapping factors combine to contribute to well being:*

Fitness. Your general health and fitness level—influenced by your weight, your diet, how much you drink and smoke, and your blood pressure—is one of the greatest contributors to longevity and to good disease prevention.

Exercise. Start off slowly, but start: You will prolong your life by increasing your heart's capacity and by strengthening your lungs and their power to circulate oxygenated blood throughout your body.

*This section has been adapted from Departmental Task Force on Prevention, *Disease Prevention and Health Promotion: Federal Programs and Prospects* (Washington, D.C.: Department of Health, Education and Welfare, Public Health Service, Office of the Assistant Secretary of Health, September 1978), DHEW publication no. (PHS) 79-55071B, p. 7; Ralph Grawunder, "How Long Will You Live Predictor," *Personal Health Appraisal,* pp. 185–91; Palmore, Erdmore, and Francis C. Jeffers, *Prediction of Life Span* (Lexington, Mass.: D. C. Heath & Co., 1971).

Emotional outlook. Your relationship with your husband or wife, your relationship with your parents, your relationship with your roommates, your ability to mix with other people, how satisfied you are with the way you live, whether your life-style is pleasant, and how well people get along with you are important contributors to good health and longevity. A positive and optimistic outlook on life coupled with a contentment with your place in life and a general satisfaction with your personal worth will make you healthier and more resistant to chronic disease.

Where you live. It makes a difference where you live. Those who live in rural areas and in small urban areas are less prone to suffer from stress that leads to heart disease and high blood pressure. Because of a myriad of factors, the state in which you live can have an effect on how long you live. Those who live in Hawaii and Utah have the longest life spans; Minnesota, North Dakota, and Wisconsin are "healthy" places to live, too. Residents of Washington, D.C., have the lowest life expectancy, followed by residents of South Carolina, Mississippi, and Louisiana.

According to *Science Digest,* the ten healthiest places to live in the United States are:

1. Any city in Hawaii
2. Eugene, Oregon
3. San Francisco, California
4. Saint Cloud, Minnesota
5. Austin, Texas
6. La Junta, Colorado
7. Utica, New York
8. Kanab, Utah
9. Ketchikan, Alaska
10. Middletown, Connecticut

On the other hand, the worst places to live, from the standpoint of health, are:

1. Washington, D.C.
2. Rhode Island
3. New Jersey
4. The entire industrialized Ohio River Valley from Wheeling, West Virginia, to Pittsburgh, Pennsylvania

5

Life-style. The unique pattern of your daily life—the food you eat, the way you get to school or work, the people you live with, the drugs you take, the cigarettes you smoke, the alcohol you drink, the hobbies you enjoy, the sports you participate in—all affect your health.

Health habits. Your health habits—whether you have a physical exam every year, whether you have a Pap smear regularly, whether you examine your breasts monthly, whether you eat three meals a day—determine what kind of health you have. Good health and longevity are linked to seven basic health habits: eating three meals a day, eating breakfast every day, exercising moderately two or three times a week, getting enough sleep, not smoking, not drinking alcohol, and keeping your weight near its ideal level.

Individual attitude. The way you look at things can play a major part in what your health is like. Laughing, believing in a religious faith, loving others, and your attitude toward yourself are important determinants of good health and well-being.

Nutrition. Eating the right things—stocking your body with the essential proteins, minerals, and vitamins—leads to good health. A machine that isn't properly fueled and well oiled can't be expected to perform at its peak. Nutrition is the basic building block that contributes to your body's well-being.

Education. People who are well educated are healthier because they have a basic understanding of the rules of sanitation, immunization, nutrition, and other health maintenance practices. The poor health that runs rampant in some underdeveloped countries is nothing but ignorance—sometimes about things as simple as washing hands after going to the bathroom.

Employment. Your employment determines how healthy you are because it can introduce environmental hazards you'd probably never encounter otherwise. You may be forced to work with asbestos, for instance, or you may spend fourteen hours a day breathing in fine particles of coal dust. Or you may sit in a soft chair behind a desk where your only exercise may be pushing a pencil.

Environment. Your environment in general—social, economic, and physical—influences your health. The water you drink and the air you breathe need to be clean; you need to enjoy your relationships with friends and family members; you need to have financial resources to meet your nutritional needs.

Psychological makeup and intelligence. You will be healthy if you can, most of the time, avoid getting depressed, avoid being bored, and avoid being under too much stress. Those who have a high regard for their own health and physical well-being, who use their mental abilities, who challenge themselves intellectually, and who are psychiatrically sound are usually healthy.

Ability to adjust. How well you can adjust to meet changing circumstances in your own life determines to a large extent your level of health.

Others. Other factors that lead to good health include good driving, healthy sexual relationships, balanced family development, ability to manage stress, and the management of risk factors that lead to disease development.

DISEASE RISK FACTORS

Currently, the top ten killers in the United States are, in order, heart disease, cancer, stroke, accidents, influenza and pneumonia, diabetes, cirrhosis of the liver, arteriosclerosis, diseases of infancy, and suicide. Although each of them is different in exact cause and in development, there are some risk factors that combine to lead to any of these killers. (Remember: A risk factor indicates whether you are more likely to get a particular disease than someone who does not have that risk factor; simply having any of the risk factors does *not* mean you will get the disease or develop the condition.)

Heredity. Of course, you can't control your heredity, but you can be alert to conditions you may develop because of heredity, and you can take what steps you can to prevent or lessen the severity of the condition. Certain diseases and dispositions toward diseases seem to be inherited—including heart disease, stroke, cancer, phlebitis, embolisms, pneumonia, tuberculosis, aneurysms, Parkinson's disease, Chiari's syndrome, and some diseases of the liver. Some forms of anemia, such as sickle-cell anemia, are also hereditary.

But wait! Remember—just because you inherit the tendency toward a condition does not mean you're helpless. You don't have to sit around glumly, waiting for the inevitable to strike. You have the responsibility to find out what hereditary factors are at work on you; then you can use the information in this book to help you pinpoint potential problem areas so you can take intelligent measures to reduce your risk and prevent trouble.

Obesity. Obesity is a serious health problem, both physically and emotionally. The physical side of the problem is critical. Each pound of fat requires three-fifths of a mile of new blood vessels to support it; a person who is thirty pounds overweight requires his cardiovascular system to construct eighteen miles of new blood vessels and requires his heart to pump blood consistently over the extra distance. It's a simple problem of overload.

7

As you'll read later, obesity is a major contributing factor to most serious diseases. It is directly responsible for eight of the ten leading causes of death—all but accidents and suicide. In some cases, it may be an indirect cause of an accident or suicide, too.

High blood pressure. When the pumping effort of the heart is increased because of high blood pressure, the heart enlarges and damage occurs to the arteries. When damage is to the arteries in the brain, stroke results; when arteries in the eyes are damaged, loss of vision can result; damaged arteries in the kidneys lead to loss of function and kidney failure.

One of the most common causes of high blood pressure is overweight. A particular cause is too much table salt. Both of these are factors you can control.

Smoking. The facts are in. Among men who have lung cancer, those who smoke have an 88 percent higher mortality rate than those who do not smoke; women smokers have a 28 percent higher mortality rate from lung cancer than women who do not smoke. The incidence of lung cancer among women has doubled in the last ten years; 80 percent of all lung cancer is directly attributable to smoking.

Smoking causes other diseases, too—and it makes many more diseases even worse.

Age. Depending on your age, you run a higher risk for developing certain conditions. Arthritis, for example, strikes people of all ages, but is much more common after middle age due to wear and tear on joints. One in four heart attack deaths occurs before the age of sixty-five. Children and young adults are more prone to accidents and suicide.

Race. Members of some racial groups run higher risks in some areas. Blacks, for example, are twice as likely as members of any other racial group to develop high blood pressure. Blacks, too, are the only racial group susceptible to sickle-cell anemia.

Stress. Stress has long been recognized as a leading cause of heart disease, but only recently have medical researchers linked stress as a major cause or contributing factor of a number of diseases—including cancer and the common cold.

Alcohol. Alcohol is now considered to be our nation's number-one drug problem; alcoholism has become a crippling disease that affects more than 19 million Americans. Ingestion of alcohol—sometimes in only moderate amounts —leads to pneumonia, cirrhosis of the liver, birth defects, and a breakdown of the body's ability to resist disease. Alcohol is frequently implicated in motor vehicle accidents, homicide, and suicide as well.

High serum cholesterol levels. Cholesterol—one of the two principal blood fats—is generally high in people who eat excessive animal fats (especially low-density fats from liver, pork, lamb, and dark fowl) and dairy products (cheese and eggs). If your blood cholesterol content is high, you run a much greater risk of developing stroke, heart disease, or vascular disease.

Diabetes. If you have diabetes, you run the risk of developing a number of other conditions, including heart disease and tuberculosis. Other general risk factors that lead to development of disease include chronic fatigue, frequent infection, lack of exercise, and electrocardiogram abnormalities.

ASSESSING RISK

What's the benefit of learning risk factors as they relate to diseases and disease conditions? The good news here is that you can do a great deal to make sure that you stay healthy.

Remember the faded embroidered sampler hanging on your grandmother's wall, the letters that spelled out "An ounce of prevention is worth a pound of cure"? That's what this book is all about. You can take an active part in preventing disease. You no longer have to wait around helplessly until disease strikes; you have the capability to define your weaknesses, to discover what diseases you might be prone to. You have the capability of defining your own risk factors—of finding out what habits, life-styles, and things in your background make you susceptible to certain diseases. And then you can do something about it!

Some diseases may involve a single significant risk. Polio, for instance, involves the risk of not being immunized. Most diseases, however, involve many contributing factors resulting from many risks; heart disease is related to people who are at risk because they are under too much stress, they smoke, they drink alcohol, they are overweight, they eat too many animal fats, they don't exercise enough, or they have uncontrolled high blood pressure.

In assessing your own risks as you read and study this book, keep in mind that a single risk factor—such as being overweight—can combine differently with other risk factors and other conditions to result in different kinds of diseases. Also keep in mind that just because you have a risk factor does not mean you will definitely develop a disease—it just means that you are one step farther toward identifying your risk of developing that disease and a whole lot closer to preventing your development of that disease. You can—and should—use your risk factors to your advantage in creating a level of wellness.

LIMITATIONS OF RISK ANALYSIS

Every person is born with a hereditary endowment that affects his maximum longevity. No one can predict exactly what your potential genetic life span will be, but we do know that acquired risk factors (including accidents) can shorten that life span.

In assessing your own risk factors, keep in mind the fact that you probably can't add many years to your own hereditary potential—you can't add many years to your life span. But you *can* eliminate the factors that may subtract years from the maximum potential that is available to you.[5]

EMPHASIS ON PREVENTION

A report issued from the Surgeon General's Office in 1980 pinpoints prevention as the single most important factor that will lead to better health for Americans everywhere. If we identify our priorities and keep a sharp focus on what we can do to reduce our own risks, the goal of prevention is attainable and possible.

THE ROLE OF THE INDIVIDUAL
The edict released from the Surgeon General's Office stated:

. . . the health of this Nation's citizens can be significantly improved through actions individuals can take themselves, and through actions decision makers in the public and private sectors can take to promote a safe and healthier environment for all Americans at home, at work, and at play. For the individual often only modest lifestyle changes are needed to substantially reduce risk for several diseases. And many of the personal decisions required to reduce risk for one disease can reduce it for others. Within the practical grasp of most Americans are simple measures to enhance the prospects of good health.[6]

What the good news boils down to is this: You can control how healthy you are.

You are responsible for your health. The most tragic health situation in this country today is that too many people neglect their own health, surrendering to someone (a doctor, a nurse, a folk healer) the complete responsibility for keeping their body well and functioning. Of course, there are many times when you must see a doctor; it would be stupid to attempt to treat yourself for what might be a serious health problem requiring medical care, for that, too, constitutes neglect. The ideal situation is an intelligent partnership with your doctor—knowing when you need help, accepting and following directions, and taking what measures you can to stay healthy.

You are responsible for being in tune with your body, for knowing when medical help is needed, for making an appointment with a doctor, for following instructions. You are the one who is responsible for following through with treatment, for taking your prescription until it is gone, for walking around the block twice a day.

THE CONCEPT OF WELLNESS

Now there is more: *You are responsible for keeping yourself well.* You have the ability to identify the things you are doing now that will shorten your life span; you have the ability to change the things you can and the intelligence to adapt to the things you can't change.

You are in control of your body and all the things that affect it.

This book is about staying well. Specifically, it's about *you* staying well. Every chapter is packed with information about how you can cope with changes that take place in your body. Every chapter is loaded with tips on how to care for yourself and prevent disease. Every chapter helps you identify your own personal risks.

REFERENCES

¹Julius B. Richmond, *Healthy People: The Surgeon General's Report on Health Promotion and Disease Prevention, 1979* (Washington, D.C.: U.S. Department of Health, Education and Welfare, Public Health Service, Office of the Assistant Secretary for Health and Surgeon General), DHEW publication no. (PHS) 79-55071, pp. v, 3.

²Ibid., p. v.

³Ibid., p. 6.

⁴Ibid.

⁵Irving S. Wright, "Can Your Family History Tell You Anything About Your Chances for a Long Life?" *Executive Health,* 14, no. 5 (February 1978), 2–3.

⁶Richmond, *Healthy People,* p. 10.

STRESS

"That scared the life right out of me!" . . . *"He makes me sick."* . . . *"The accident took ten years off my life!"* . . . *"She gives me a pain in the neck."*

Meaningless sayings? No.

A frightening experience, one that evokes severe enough emotions, can cause death. Facing a person who leads us to feel rejected or who causes us to feel uncomfortable can make us sick (most often causing respiratory problems or the common cold). The stress caused by an accident can age you. Dealing with an unpleasant person can cause neck pains.

It all has to do with stress—with the way our bodies react to physical, chemical, or emotional changes.[1] Those changes—physical, emotional, or chemical—cause physical or emotional tension, otherwise known as *stress*.

Each of us is under stress all of the time. Some stress is relatively minor (did I remember to put a nickel in the parking meter? did I unplug the iron before I left the house?), while some stress is severe (will I lose my job over that bad report? is my wife going to die from complications of her surgery? is my husband going to file for divorce?). All stress—whether minor or severe—has an effect on your body. Stress is, literally, the response of the body to any demand that is made upon the body.[2]

Once it's under stress, the body reacts—physiologically as well as emotionally—to try and normalize things again. The wear and tear of stress takes its toll: As many as 80 percent of all people who go to doctors do so because of stress-related illnesses.[3] In fact, some doctors think that *all* illnesses, at least in part, are caused by stress.

None of us could survive in an environment totally free of stress, either. A group of athletes were forced to lie on their beds for two weeks; none could

12

engage in any activity at all. Their internal organs and their circulatory systems began to suffer lower performance levels; at the end of the two weeks their muscles had started to soften and their bones had started to deteriorate.[4] The key, then, rests in learning to cope effectively with stress and in taking measures to reduce stress when it becomes severe.

WHAT CAUSES STRESS?

Because each of us is an individual, each of us reacts differently to different situations, and each of us experiences stress as a result of different things.

Stress can result from negative things—such as divorce, death, or illness —but it can also be the result of positive things—such as getting married, winning an athletic contest, receiving a promotion at work, being recognized for an outstanding achievement. Your mind can distinguish between "positive" (or "good") and "negative" (or "bad") situations and stresses, but your body can't: Your body reacts the same way to positive as to negative stress.

Sometimes simply *anticipating* a stressful situation (such as taking an exam or going to the dentist) can, in itself, produce tension. This kind of anticipation is what caused you to lie awake all night before you started your new job or before you competed in the golf tournament.

Even though each individual reacts to stress in a different way, doctors and researchers have been able to isolate some events that seem universally to cause stress. These include everything from the death of a spouse to Christmas.[5]

Many causes of stress are unavoidable. You can't control your mother's death from leukemia, nor can you prevent an earthquake that destroys your small town and necessitates a move to a nearby city during reconstruction. Other causes of stress *are* avoidable, though: if you get nervous and upset in crowds, avoid them. Do your Christmas shopping early, and watch the football game on television instead of fighting the crowd at the stadium. If violent movies cause you a great deal of upset, don't go to them. Avoid stress where you can, and it will be easier for you to cope in those instances when you *can't* avoid stress.

Review the list of factors that are known to cause stress at the end of this chapter. Think of ways that you can reduce your own stress. For instance, if you recently got married and your wife is pregnant, you would probably be better off not buying a house right away—especially if buying the house would mean moving to a different town or assuming a large mortgage. If you were recently divorced, think twice before you change your job, move to a new community, go back to school, or enter a new relationship that might involve sexual intimacies —all situations that can add significantly to the stress of the divorce.

Your occupation can have a great deal to do with the amount of stress you suffer, too.[6] Jobs with exceptionally high levels of stress include factory laborer, secretary, inspector, clinical laboratory technician, office manager, foreman, manager/administrator, waitress/waiter, machine operator, farm owner, mine operative, painter (not artist), machinist, mechanic, structural metal craftsperson, plumber, electrician, meat cutter, salesperson, public relations person, policeman/policewoman, fireman, member of the clergy, social worker, therapist, nurse, nurse's aide, hospital orderly, health aide, dental assistant, and health technician.

People in some occupations suffer very few stress-related disorders; those occupations include sewer worker, examiner or checker, stockhandler, craftsperson, maid, farm laborer, heavy equipment operator, freight handler, packer or wrapper, child care worker, college or university professor, labor relations person, personnel administrator, and auctioneer or huckster.[7]

What affects how much stress is caused by a certain occupation? A great deal of stress results when workers have too much or too little to do, when a job is too difficult or too easy for a worker's level of skill, when a job is unstable because of reorganization or other changeable factors, when a worker is presented with conflicting demands (either from two different superiors or from both a superior and fellow workers), when a worker is responsible for other people (such as a foreman, who is responsible for all the workers on his crew), when a worker does not have the opportunity of making decisions that affect his or her job, when the job requires a great deal of concentration (such as wiring microscopic components on an assembly line), when a worker is a subject of unequal pay, or when a worker does not enjoy the social support of fellow workers or supervisors. In short, it's the people who have a lot of responsibility but little authority—such as the nurse who works under a staff of doctors—or who have a lot of responsibility but little control—such as the worker on an assembly line, who can't control whether it goes or stops—who suffer from the highest amount of stress.

Workers who can derive a high sense of satisfaction from their jobs—such as family doctors, university professors, company officials—rate low on the stress scale because they tend to have more sources of satisfaction than the workers listed in the foregoing examples.

HOW DOES THE BODY
REACT TO STRESS?

Whenever it is threatened in any way, the body prepares for the "fight." In a strict medical sense, stress is anything that triggers the body's adaptive mechanisms, anything that helps the body get ready to protect itself by causing these mechanisms, or reactions, to occur.[8] These reactions, which enable us to cope with stress or to meet a stressful situation, are the same reactions that enable us to run from an approaching automobile that is about to run us over, to fight off an attacker, to chase a bus, to lift a fallen tree off the body of a young child.

Physical reactions to stress—reactions that prepare the body for a fight—include the following:

1. The cerebral cortex, located in the brain, sends impulses along a complicated network of nerves that interact to create a state of preparedness in the body.
2. The heart pumps faster and with stronger beats, circulating the blood more efficiently to provide additional fuel for the body.
3. Skeletal muscles, especially those required for quick motion or for lifting or pushing, contract and become filled with oxygenated blood, preparatory for motion.
4. The spleen contracts, forcing increased blood circulation.
5. Eyesight is sharpened due to impulses sent from the cerebral cortex along the optic nerve.
6. The sense of smell is sharpened, due to impulses sent from the cerebral cortex along the olfactory nerve.
7. The adrenal glands are stimulated, causing the secretion of large amounts of adrenaline.
8. Blood vessels in the skin are stimulated to contract, resulting in a reddening of the skin (especially in the facial area, causing a flushing of the face during extreme fear or anger).
9. Further stimulation of the adrenal glands, especially the adrenal medulla, causes a heightening of blood sugar, resulting in a quick burst of energy.
10. The airways leading to the lungs and the air passages in the lungs dilate, allowing for deep breathing necessary in vigorous physical activity.
11. The pupils are dilated.
12. Chemicals released in the skeletal muscles act to reduce muscle fatigue and allow the muscles to sustain long-term rigorous activity without giving out.
13. Chemicals reduced into the bloodstream accelerate the coagulating function of the blood (if the body is injured, the blood will clot much more rapidly).
14. Nerve impulses sent from the cerebral cortex along the pelvic nerve (sacral parasympathetic nerve) signal the bladder to evacuate—which is why some people lose control of their bladder during extreme fear.

These reactions on the part of the body enable a person to lash out at or escape from an attacker—enable him or her to see and smell more acutely, to keep punching or running for a longer period of time, to breathe more rapidly, to avoid bleeding severely from an injury. But a person who has just been told that he or she did not get an expected pay raise goes through much the same physical reaction—with no way to vent rage, no way to express the body's preparedness. People who have no avenue of physical expression undergo tremendous wear and tear on their bodies.

SIGNS OF STRESS

Various signs—both physical and mental—can signal the onset of stress. Physical symptoms of stress include

- increased cholesterol level in the blood (detected by laboratory results)
- high blood pressure
- rapid pulse
- loss of appetite
- tendency to overeat (especially in response to stressful situations)
- queasiness in the stomach ("butterflies")
- nausea
- heartburn
- eyestrain
- fluttering motions of the eyes
- tightened muscles in the neck and jaw
- grinding of the teeth
- clenching of the jaw
- cold hands
- sweating palms
- excessive sweating elsewhere on the body
- contraction and tightness of general body muscles
- jerky movement
- irregular or shallow breathing
- strained voice, often becoming high-pitched
- hunching posture (resulting from excessive tightening of shoulder muscles)
- rigid spine, preventing fluid movement
- tight forehead muscles, causing change in facial expression

- contraction of muscles in fingers and toes, causing them to curl
- headache
- twitching and trembling
- dryness of mouth
- lack of interest in sex
- frigidity
- impotence
- menstrual disorders
- nervousness, including the tendency to be frightened or startled easily
- excessive belching
- chronic diarrhea
- chronic constipation
- chronic indigestion (including belching, heartburn, and nausea)
- weakness and fatigue
- dizziness
- tendency to faint easily
- fainting spells preceded by nausea
- difficulty in falling asleep
- inability to remain asleep during the night
- inability to sit still
- tendency to tire easily
- muscle spasms
- feeling of fullness without eating
- inability to cry
- tendency to burst into tears at slight provocation or for no reason at all

Mental symptoms of stress include

- depression
- irritability
- the desire to escape from people or things or situations
- strong urge to cry
- impulsive behavior that is incompatible with normal patterns of behavior
- feelings of anxiety, sometimes vague or ill defined
- inability to think clearly
- inability to make simple decisions

- inability to solve simple problems
- lack of desire to participate fully in life
- feelings of self-destruction
- impatience
- tendency to be extremely critical of others
- meticulousness about surroundings and possessions
- tendency to be a perfectionist
- tendency to lose temper
- inability to relax physically
- feelings of mild panic
- frustration and concern over health (especially worries over minor aches and pains)
- fear of death
- fear of disease (especially cancer)
- fear of insanity or mental illness
- fear of being alone
- inability to cope with criticism
- inability to get along with others
- inability to concentrate
- feeling of separation or removal from people and things once important and vital
- tendency to live mostly in the past
- boredom
- feeling of inability to cope with problems and frustrations
- inability to freely express emotion, especially anger
- feeling of rejection by family members
- feeling of failure as a parent
- inability to confide problems or concerns in another person

In some instances stress is short-lived; the stress-provoking situation is removed or is resolved, and you are able to move on without feeling many ill effects from your bout with stress. In other instances, however, the stress is of extreme duration (sometimes a lifetime, such as a person who is born without arms or legs, or sometimes for many years, such as the young man or woman who divorces early in marriage and who never remarries). In those situations, the ongoing stress literally *wears out* the body. One of the most significant ways that it wears out the body, of course, is by causing disease.

WHO IS MOST PRONE
TO STRESS?

As stated earlier, each person is an individual, different from every other person, so each person reacts differently to stress-promoting factors in his or her life. Some people, however, are much more prone than others to cope poorly with stress; these people have several personality factors in common. Others, because of their personality traits, are better able to deal with stress.

Researchers have divided the human race into two general personality types:[9]

TYPE-A PERSONALITY

Type-A people, those who are much more likely to develop a stress-related problem or illness, are characterized by the following behavioral patterns:

- They are extremely competitive.
- They are schedule and time oriented, and they tend to make schedules and lists of activities for themselves.
- They are extremely concerned with success and with social acceptance.
- They are numbers oriented: They like to *count* their successes, achievements, and possessions.
- They move and speak quickly; they sometimes forget to finish their sentences, and if someone else hesitates midsentence, they are apt to finish the sentence for the faltering person.
- They like to set several goals at once for themselves; they are rarely content with working on just one project at a time. They are strictly punctual, and they are intolerant of others who are late to appointments and meetings.
- They are extremely concerned about coming out on top; if they participate in a competitive or sports event of any kind, they must win.
- They are compulsively meticulous about their surroundings and their possessions.
- They are easily upset by others.
- They are hostile and aggressive toward those whom they perceive as competition.
- They set unrealistic goals for themselves.

In conclusion, type-A people not only lack the ability to cope adequately with stress—they *create* stress for themselves by the way that they live and through behavior patterns. Medical researchers have isolated the type-A personality as the one exhibiting behavior patterns that consistently lead to heart disease.

But these natural pushers and go-getters—these people with an overabundance of ambition and drive—suffer. The classical career pattern of type-A people goes something like this: They pace themselves early, rise quickly through the ranks, experience real success or achievement early in their careers, experience a high level of involvement, and then crash. Why?

Because their minds and bodies can't keep up with the pace. The amount of stress they have suffered in their rise to the top has literally torn up their bodies. They are exhausted and depressed.

Once this stress-induced exhaustion sets in, they lose interest in activities outside of work. They are unable to enjoy activities and interests away from their jobs, but their enjoyment in their jobs disappears, too. They have to try harder, and even then they can't seem to achieve what they did before. They alternate between periods of dark pessimism and wild optimism. Suddenly they replace effort and work with the search for a shortcut, a magic solution. They become suspicious of their colleagues, who seem hostile; and they devote their time and energy to criticizing them.

Before long, they develop physical problems that go along with their mental ones. They get headaches, muscle spasms, lethargy; unfortunately, their reaction is to eat more. They get even more sluggish.

Because type-A people have a difficult time relaxing, they resort to cigarette smoking or to drinking to try to unwind. Type-A people are more prone to accidents on the job because they have a hard time concentrating and because they try to achieve results and finish tasks more quickly.

Basically, the type-A person is in a hurry.

TYPE-B PERSONALITY

Type-B people, those who are better able to cope with stress partly because they create less stress for themselves, are characterized by the following behavioral patterns:

- They are easygoing.
- They are seldom impatient; they are content with waiting for success, for lunch lines, for buses that are late.
- They do not worry much.
- They make their own decisions; they are generally not influenced by other people. Their decisions are not based on an attempt to gain social acceptance, career status, or professional recognition. The approval of others is not important to them.
- They are able to see things in longer perspective than a type-A person; they set longer-term goals and are content with taking a longer time to achieve goals.

- They are realistic about what they can achieve; their goals reflect this realism, and they tend to work on only one or two goals at a time.
- They are relatively unworried about the future.
- They are able to make decisions easily.
- They recognize that petty irritations are simply *petty,* and they are much less critical of others.
- They accept the fact that they cannot achieve all things at once.
- They are less concerned with schedules; if they set a deadline for themselves, they are unworried and accepting if they miss the deadline.

A type-B person is not lazy or necessarily lacking in force: A type-B person simply moves ahead through relaxation, patience, and methodical application of work techniques while the type-A person moves ahead through sheer drive and energy. A type-A person presses forward frantically, working harder and faster than a type-B person, pushing deadlines even farther ahead, jamming in more assignments, giving up more leisure time. But when a type-A person burns out, a type-B person is still methodically and patiently working toward achieving his or her goals.

Neither personality type has the corner on intelligence or ambition or position in society—each category includes company presidents, truck drivers, ditch diggers, and attorneys. But because a type-A person actually creates a greater volume of stress, he or she is much more likely to develop heart disease, high blood pressure, and diabetes. A type-A person also tends to have a higher cholesterol level and to suffer more from all diseases in general.

Some factors in your personality are beyond your control; with help, you can learn to control and overcome others. Later in this chapter techniques for relaxation and control of stress will be discussed. If you have a type-A personality, you can learn to reduce your overload of frustration and to lengthen your effective achievement span—and, most critical of all, to cope better with the stress you can't control and to eliminate the stress you can.

STRESS AND DISEASE

Disease originally meant a lack of ease—not illness.[10]

Today, that concept still holds true: Those who are not at ease—who are suffering the effects of stress—are those who are likely to sicken.

Medical researchers unraveling the puzzle of disease discovered the involvement of germs in illness but failed to solve one final, critical riddle: What causes the onset of disease? Since then we have discovered something that challenges all of our previous ideas about disease: Events of ordinary life, such as marriage, a vacation, a new job, a personal achievement, can help trigger illness, because the effort that is required to cope with these life events weakens our resistance.[11]

In other words, stress causes disease.

The results of one fascinating study serve to bear out that hypothesis. A group of patients who reported to a doctor with symptoms of a cold or nasal infection were asked to return to the same doctor when their symptoms had disappeared. As each patient returned to the doctor, the doctor measured the patient's freedom of breathing, amount of swelling in the nasal passages, amount of secretion in the nose, and blood flow. Each was pronounced recovered. The doctor then started to talk to the patient about the event or events that occurred just prior to the onset of the illness—his or her acceptance of a new position with the company, the week-long visit of his or her mother-in-law, or the death of a close friend, for example. Then the doctor repeated the same physiological tests.

Amazingly, the cold symptoms had returned. By simply *talking about* the stress-provoking situations, the doctor had caused a recurrence of a disease in a completely healthy person! Nasal tissue biopsies confirmed that actual tissue damage had occurred during the discussion of the stressful situation.[12]

Stress—feelings of anxiety, hostility, and conflict—brings about actual physical changes, as discussed earlier. It can alter body chemistry and organ function, but if we are in good health and living a well-balanced life-style, we have the capacity to restore ourselves to a state of equilibrium. In other words, if we're in good shape physically and emotionally, we can bounce back easily from periods of brief stress without feeling any ill effects.[13]

What happens when the stress is severe, prolonged, inescapable, or intensified? Or what happens if we are not in good health physically and/or emotionally? Just the opposite: The stress causes very real and severe harm to us, both physically and emotionally. Our body's efforts to normalize itself are frustrated, and disease and illness may result.

PAIN

Pain, a sensory signal indicating that the body's state of normality is being threatened or disrupted, is perceived in much the same way as sights, sounds, smells, and tastes are perceived.[14] It involves the stimulation of nerves, and it is accompanied by an emotional response of varying magnitudes.[15]

Stress affects not only the development of pain but the perception of pain. A person who is rigid, goal oriented, and forceful in personality—a type-A person—will perceive pain as being more intense than will a more easygoing person (a type-B person). Pain that may practically render a type-A person as a bed-bound invalid may merely be noticed and tolerated by a type-B person.

There are physiological changes as well. When the body is under stress, the chemical responsible for lowering the pain threshold cannot be retained by normal blood platelets, and the victim perceives pain more intensely.[16] In addition, the chronic depression that is a result of severe stress has been shown to be the precursor to most chronic pain conditions.

STRESS AND SUDDEN DEATH

Overwhelming stress—generally that caused by deep personal losses (such as death of a spouse), situations involving personal danger, or situations involving intense relief—that is impossible to ignore, that evokes intense emotions, and that is beyond an individual's control can and does cause sudden death.[17]

Several factors are responsible for the phenomenon of sudden death due to stress:

Hopelessness. In an experiment a laboratory rat was dumped into a tank of water; it struggled and thrashed around, swimming for almost sixty hours before it finally drowned. A second rat was held in the experimenter's hand for a few minutes; the experimenter curled his fingers tightly around the rat as if to strangle or suffocate it. The rat struggled against the experimenter for several minutes before finally going limp. The rat was then dumped into the same tank of water; it struggled for less than two minutes before sinking to the bottom and dying.

Why was there such a difference in the reaction between the two rats once they hit the water?

The second rat had already given up hope of survival. It was suffering from the stress that accompanies hopelessness, and that stress rendered it incapable of fighting for its life.

The same applies to human beings: Those who have "given up" or who determine that they are in a helpless or hopeless situation undergo actual physical changes that lead to death. Sudden death can also occur in those who struggle incessantly (in a job, family situation, or social context) without experiencing satisfaction or success.[18]

Prediction of death. People under stress who decide that they are going to die—such as patients who face a surgical operation—often experience a predilection to death: They predict their own deaths. For some who are burdened with excessive stress death is viewed as a welcome escape from problems and pain, and death actually does occur within an extremely brief period of time.

Life changes. Stress-provoking life changes (as listed in Part I of the Self-Evaluation Test at the end of this chapter), such as death of a spouse, marriage, divorce, foreclosure of a mortgage, or loss of a job, can result in

23

sudden death due to the body's inability to accommodate the changes that occur in the cardiovascular system. As discussed earlier, stress causes physiological changes, among them a pounding of the heart, rapid circulation of the blood, and constriction of the arteries and vessels leading to skeletal muscles. When the body cannot tolerate these reactions to severe stress, heart attack results, and sudden death is the end result of the stress situation.

Hypertension. High blood pressure is a well-documented effect of prolonged and severe stress and can also occur after a brief period of intense or unexpected stress. If it is severe enough, hypertension due to stress can result in death.

Cardiac rhythms. Because stress clearly affects the heart's rhythm, cardiac arrhythmias that accompany sudden and long-term intensified stress can cause sudden death.

Myocardial necrosis. Long-term stress that cannot be resolved by the physical systems of the body results in chemical secretions that actually cause deterioration of the heart muscle, leading to sudden and unexpected death.

Arteriosclerosis. Disease and damage involving the coronary arteries is a common result of prolonged or intense stress and can result in myocardial infarction, leading to sudden death.

The dive reflex. A reflex that occurs when you dive into a pool full of water—the heart slows down, blood flow to the skin and internal organs is reduced, arterial blood pressure is increased, blood pH is reduced, lactic acid is increased, carbon dioxide in the blood increases, and potassium levels in the blood increase—can also occur as a result of severe stress (either long-term or sudden). If these physiological changes are not promptly corrected—as they are when a diver returns to the surface of the water—sudden death results.

DECREASED IMMUNITY TO DISEASE

Because they affect the function of the body's immunologic system as a result of their effects on the central nervous system, stress and distress impair the body's ability to resist disease.*

*This section adapted from George F. Solomon, "Emotions, Stress, the Central Nervous System, and Immunity," *Annals of the New York Academy of Sciences*, 164 (1969), 335–42; George L. Engel, "The Psychosomatic Approach to Individual Susceptibility to Disease," *Gastroenterology*, 67 (1974), 1085–93.

Disease is a result of several factors working together: The presence of bacteria, virus, or some other disease-causing element; host tissue in the body that can be affected by the disease-causing element (such as lungs that can be inflamed by a tuberculosis bacteria); and some internal or external factor that lowers the body's resistance to the disease-causing factor. Stress—particularly stress severe enough to result in depression—can lower the body's ability to resist disease and infection. This decreased immunity can make the body susceptible to communicable diseases of all kinds and to certain other diseases, such as heart disease, respiratory illness, and cancer.

HEART DISEASE

A number of risk factors lead to the development of heart disease; among them are cigarette smoking, high blood cholesterol levels, obesity, lack of exercise, diabetes, family history and genetic makeup, and age.* But physical factors alone will not determine that a person will develop heart disease or will die from a heart attack: The determining factor is his ability to cope with stress.

Prime candidates for heart attack and heart disease are the type-A personalities—people who are highly competitive, who feel pressured for time, who set deadlines and quotas for themselves, who feel frustrated when they can't meet their impossibly high goals, and who react to frustration with hostility. Type-A people are the prime candidates because they create stress for themselves and because their high levels of stress interfere with their bodies' ability to return to a normal state of affairs.

Other causes of heart disease and heart attack are the stresses that accompany such life changes as a deep personal loss, a change in environment, a move to a new community, or a demotion in a job.

Stress causes the following physical changes, all of which can lead to heart disease and heart attack:

1. Cholesterol levels in the bloodstream are increased; these cholesterol deposits adhere to the walls of the arteries, causing a narrowing and hardening of the arteries.
2. Blood is sent coursing through the arteries at a high pressure, causing hypertension.
3. Fatty deposits formed from cholesterol and plaque break away from the artery walls, traveling through the bloodstream and lodging in the heart, lung, or brain, causing death. The deposits tear away in response to stress and its effect on the pressure of the bloodstream.

*This section adapted from David C. Glass, "Stress, Competition, and Heart Attacks," *Psychology Today*, December 1976, pp. 55–57.

4. Physiological changes that occur as a result of stress increase the body's blood-clotting mechanism, causing the blood to thicken and clot in the small arteries and possibly lead to death.

RESPIRATORY ILLNESS

The greater the intensity of stress, the greater the likelihood that disease will develop and that it will be serious enough to cripple or kill.* Respiratory illnesses—especially tuberculosis, asthma, sore throat, the common cold, and hay fever—have been positively linked to stress and its effects on the body.

Three kinds of stress seem to precipitate respiratory illness:

1. Failure and disappointment (which lead to a sense of personal helplessness and hopelessness).
2. Separation from family and friends or a modification in the relationship with family and friends.
3. Rising status and positive achievement.

People suffering from depression that tends to overwhelm or frighten them are especially high risk in relation to respiratory illness. In relation to such stress-involved depression, four factors seem to cause serious respiratory illness:

1. A sense of impending failure or an actual failure in an aspect of life that is important to the individual. (For instance, a woman who prides herself on being a good mother may develop an acute case of asthma serious enough to require hospitalization if her neglect results in her child being struck and killed by an automobile.)
2. A sense of helplessness to change what happens as a result of the failure. (This same mother, for example, cannot restore life to her child, nor can she reverse the chain of events that led to the child's death.)
3. The feeling that one is responsible for the failure. (The mother may decide that she is to blame because when she went into town to run errands, she left the child in the care of another child who was too young to baby-sit. If only she had taken her child with her or had left her under adult supervision . . .)
4. A sense of being isolated and without support. (The mother may feel an

*This section adapted from Martin A. Jacobs, Aron Z. Spilken, Martin M. Norman, and Luleen S. Anderson, "Life Stress and Respiratory Illness," *Psychosomatic Medicine,* 32 no. 3 (May–June 1970), 233–42; Aman U. Khan, "Present Status of Psychosomatic Aspects of Asthma," *Psychosomatics,* July–August 1973, pp. 195–200; Thomas J. Luparello, "When Emotional Conflict Complicates Respiratory Disease," *Medical Insight,* April 1971, pp. 22–35.

overwhelming sense of grief and may decide that others around her—her husband, her other children, the neighbors—can't really understand what she is going through because none of them has lost a child in such a tragic manner, even though her husband lost the same child.)

The more severe and intense the stress invoked by the sense of failure and helplessness, the more severe the disease that results and the greater the likelihood of death.

CANCER

Although they do not yet understand the exact physiological reasons, medical researchers recently concluded that stress may influence the development of cancer; the most probable explanation is the tendency of stress to reduce the body's ability to fight disease in general.* Stress's effect on the body's immunology and endocrinology is probably what leads to the development of concern and other malignant diseases.

As with other illnesses and diseases, cancer seems to be precipitated by certain conditions. Among these are severe, stress-induced depression, a sense of hopelessness, and a deep personal loss resulting in stress. In addition, researchers have discovered that there is a distinct "cancer personality"—much as there is a personality prone to heart disease—that of a type-A person. Basic to this personality is the overriding stress and anxiety that lead to depression. Many cancer victims also have stress-induced spells of confusion, disorientation, and phobia.

Of special interest was a recent study of women who developed cancer of the breast or cervix. Those developing cancer of the breast commonly suffered from depression and guilt; common to women who developed cancer of the cervix was a disturbance over sexual activities and a guilt related to sexual performance or activity. Most of the women were disturbed about their identities as women and had a history of excessive responsibility during childhood.

OTHER DISEASES

A number of diseases are related directly to the amount of stress created by life-style. Stress ulcers—both gastric and duodenal—have long been identified with stress and anxiety and are a result of the physiological changes created in the body in response to stress, including the excretion of excess digestive acids and the secretion of hormones that lead to tissue destruction. Migraine headache,

*This section adapted from Frida G. Surawicz, Dennis R. Brightwell, William D. Weitzel, and Ekkehard Othmer, "Cancer, Emotions, and Mental Illness: The Present State of Understanding," *American Journal of Psychiatry,* 133, no. 11 (November 1976), 1306–9.

tension headache, colitis, loss of teeth (due to grinding and chemical damage to the gums), gum disease, growth of extra teeth, chronic low back pain, and a number of childhood diseases may be attributed to stress and to the body's inability to cope with stress by returning its systems to normal.

PSYCHOSOMATIC ILLNESS AND HYPOCHONDRIA

You've probably heard the terms *psychosomatic illness* and *hypochondriac,* and you may have confused the two: Stan's ulcer is actually a psychosomatic illness, the doctor said, and Maren's ulcer is due to the fact that she is a hypochondriac. So Stan's illness and Maren's illness are actually the same, right?

Wrong.

We are actually made up of two components: a physical body and a mind (or spirit). Many people regard the two to be one unit; others deal with the mind and the body as separate entities requiring separate treatment and consideration.

Whether you consider the mind and body to be separate or united, you should realize that the mind has powerful effects on the body. Stress, in fact, is a product of the mind working on the body—it's a process of the mind prompting the body to become prepared for an emergency or a situation requiring excess strength and action.

Psychosomatic is a term derived from the words *psyche,* meaning "mind," and *soma,* meaning "body." A psychosomatic disease, then, is a disease that results from the mind's influence over the body. A psychosomatic disease is caused by the mind, but the symptoms are very real. A psychosomatically induced ulcer, for instance, is an actual open sore in the stomach lining; a psychosomatically induced heart attack involves actual tissue destruction to the heart and irregularity in the heart's rhythm—it can even cause death.

Hypochondriacs, on the other hand, *think* they are ill. But they are not. They may experience extreme discomfort after they eat, may suffer from heartburn, and may have sharp abdominal pains—all the classic symptoms of ulcer. Upon examination, however, even a test including X-ray examinations, the hypochondriac patient's stomach is verified to be completely normal. Hypochondriacs may suffer all the symptoms of any one of a hundred diseases, but laboratory tests will always come back negative. They have no illness.

That's where the difference lies: The hypochondriac's illness is all in his or her head, while the psychosomatic illness is simply *caused* by the head. A hypochondriac's stomach lining is healthy and unmarred; a psychosomatically induced ulcer patient has an ulcerated stomach lining that is aggravated by excess stomach acid and that may even bleed.

28

As mentioned earlier in this chapter, doctors now believe that all illnesses may be caused in part by stress—by the way we react to stressors in our environment. So, all diseases and illnesses might be considered, at least partially, as psychosomatically induced. But that's a far cry from considering all of us to be hypochondriacs!

COPING WITH STRESS

While there are some things we simply cannot change—the death of a spouse who was killed in an airplane accident or the bursting of a dam that floods the community and washes our priceless possessions down the river—there are things we can change and things we can do to cope with stress and to lessen its effects on us and on our bodies.

BIOFEEDBACK

Each human being has certain rhythms within his body that regulate how he reacts and how his body functions; these rhythms are called *circadian rhythms,* and, if measured, they can tell us a great deal about ourselves and how we are managing stress and other factors in our lives.

Some researchers have recently developed the ability to measure these rhythms with the use of biofeedback machines, which give you feedback on what's going on inside. The theory is that once you are aware of how you're doing—of how your own circadian rhythms react to different stresses—you can take steps to control and change the way your body functions (again, an example of mind over matter).

What's measured by biofeedback equipment? Hand temperature. Muscle tension. Electrical brain activity. All kinds of body activities, most of which you are unconscious of under normal conditions. Biofeedback helps you become aware that your brain is emitting theta waves from the visual section, a finding that means you will probably be prone to more creative thoughts. In other words, theta wave activity tends to consist of "thoughts" translated into visual images that are not inhibited by learned experience. Therefore, the thoughts are often new, original, and thus more creative. Biofeedback helps you become aware that the muscles in your forehead are tense and rigid, a signal of unusual stress and tension. Therapists trained in biofeedback methods can help you interpret your rhythms and learn how to control stress in your own situation.

Biofeedback is only one way of managing stress. Other ways to overcome stress and to help keep its ill effects in check include:

1. Learn to relax. The actual method of relaxation depends on what works best for the individual. Some things that may be very relaxing to one person may actually induce additional stress in another. Assess ways that you can relax during the day; try taking a short nap in the afternoon, taking a fifteen-minute walk during the morning break at work, finding a quiet place to be by yourself during the day, taking a hot bath when you get home from work, massaging your feet, reading a favorite book or magazine, or taking up a hobby (such as carpentry, sewing, quilting, writing, or hiking). The important thing is to regularly spend time doing something that you enjoy and that you do not feel pressure to succeed at. You should learn to take time out of your schedule simply to sit back and take a breather—to forget about the problems that are weighing on you as a result of your job, your family, or some social situation that concerns you.

Don't choose something that you think will be good for you as a leisure time activity; choose something that you *like*. Really enjoy yourself.

2. Get enough exercise.

Exercise has all kinds of benefits; one of them is that it provides a physical release for the pent-up rage and hostility that accompanies stress. As was discussed earlier, the physical changes that your body goes through under stress are the same ones it goes through in reaction to threat or danger. When you have to ward off an attacker or run from a burning building, your body has a chance to work and to release the emotions and the physiological chemicals it has built up to prepare it for the emergency: The pounding heart helps you run; your rapid breathing helps fuel your body; your stimulated adrenal glands send adrenaline coursing through your system, enabling you to work with increased strength and endurance; and the blood-clotting properties of the body help you recover quickly from an injury. But when your body gets all keyed up in response to the news that you have been fired from your job, there isn't much you can do to express your emotions or release the physiological tension.

Exercise provides one way to help your body return to normal by working off the chemical and physical changes resulting from stress. Exercise can also help you relax by lessening the tension placed on muscles and body organs. In addition, it helps increase circulation, contributing to a sense of overall well-being. Finally, it helps develop your self-confidence and sense of accomplishment. Before beginning any exercise program, however, check with your doctor; he can instruct you as to the exercises that will best benefit you in consideration of your total general fitness, your body type, any physical disabilities you may have, and your body's tolerance level.

One important consideration: You should *like* the exercise you're doing. Exercise doesn't necessarily mean standing on a foam mat and methodically performing jumping jacks, sit-ups, push-ups, and deep knee bends—unless you like that kind of thing. Exercise can also mean playing raquetball with your best friend, swimming, playing tennis with your spouse, jogging with a group from the office, or playing basketball on the church team. Whatever kind of exercise you choose, it should provide a chance to relieve your boredom, excite your senses, and provide relaxation and fun.

Your doctor can best advise you as to the exact frequency best for you, but you should get involved in *some* kind of physical activity every day. This doesn't mean that you need to play an exhausting game of tennis doubles every day; it does mean that if you only play tennis on Saturdays, you should find something else to do on the other days. One day you might simply walk around the block; another day you might climb the stairs to your office instead of taking the elevator. You might simply decide to stretch at your desk and do some simple calisthenics.

In addition to your daily routine of mild exercise, you should engage in vigorous exercise—such as swimming, tennis, or running—at least three times a week.

3. Organize your day according to what you really want to do. This means taking a realistic look at yourself, your capabilities, and your goals. For a few days try making a list of things that you need or want to do. Look at the list and decide which things on it are absolutely crucial—eating lunch, for example—and which things you can delegate to someone else—meeting with a stubborn client about an account that you share with several other executives, for instance. Decide which things on the list will help you reach your goals—either for the day, the week, or the year—and which aren't really important. Then concentrate on the things that are necessary, that you enjoy, and that will help you achieve your goals. It is important to feel a sense of satisfaction and accomplishment, so keep your list within the bounds of what you can realistically handle; overshooting or overestimating your abilities will only lead to frustration and a sense of failure when you are unable to complete everything on your list.

4. Learn to keep crises in their places. Learn to distinguish between minor crises and major ones; you'll find, to your surprise, that most problems and crises in life are minor. When you encounter a minor problem, solve it. Then forget it.

5. Eliminate unnecessary activities from your life. Learn that life is *not* a constant struggle against the clock. Don't cut out the things that give you relaxation and enjoyment, but try to identify the things that you could delegate to someone else or that you could forget altogether. Then learn to loosen up your schedule so that you have time to do the things you do choose to do.

6. When you feel yourself getting rushed or panicked, stop. Perform some conscious slowdown maneuvers. Deep breathing is a good one. Simply sitting at your desk for a few minutes with your eyes closed and your hands lying flat on the desk top can also help. Don't resume your activities until you feel you've regained control and are not senselessly rushed.

7. Try to work in an environment that is peaceful. Most offices and other work environments have a little bit of dissension and quibbling now and then, but you should not try to keep working in an environment that is constantly in turmoil. (You might even consider quitting or asking to be transferred to another office if the problems are severe enough.) If you work in your home, take measures necessary to make your home a happy, relaxing place to live in.

8. Learn to live day by day instead of living always in the future. Pay attention to what is going on here and now; look around you and try to learn to appreciate the beauty and enjoyment available to you *now* instead of constantly driving yourself for some intangible and vague beauty and enjoyment you will be able to enjoy in the future.

9. If something is worrying you, talk it over with a trusted friend or family member. Keeping a worry bottled up inside you can only cause you to become frustrated, depressed, and even more worried. One of the most devastating results of stress is a feeling of hopelessness and helplessness. Try talking your worry over with someone else; they might be able to offer a solution you hadn't even thought of.

10. If you encounter a serious or a mild problem, escape for a brief time to give yourself a chance to collect your thoughts and calm your emotions. Go to a movie, go for a walk, play with your child, get involved in a basketball game. After a *short* escape, return to your problem and tackle it. Trying to escape permanently or for a long period of time will only serve to increase your stress and the effect it has on your body.

11. When you feel pent-up rage, frustration, or emotion of any kind, do something physically active. Rake the lawn, weed the garden, ride your bicycle to town and back, have a race with your child to the end of the block, or challenge your best friend to a quick game of tennis.

12. If you are frequently involved in quarrels and if you are usually defiant, learn to give a little. It is important that you hold your ground where principles and moral values are involved, but refusing to budge on a nonessential issue is stupid and serves to increase your stress level. Learn to compromise a little, and don't view giving in slightly as a sign of weakness or failure.

13. If you are faced with a work load that seems unbearable, divide it into a series of smaller tasks. Then tackle the tasks, one by one, until you finish the larger job. For example, when you are opening the morning mail at your office, open each letter, read it, and act on it before you open the next one. Don't sit and read through the whole pile, stacking it haphazardly on your desk, and feeling inadequate and unable to cope with it when you are through opening envelopes.

14. Don't try to be perfect in everything you do. You are a human being and are therefore subject to frailty and error. You should give your best effort to everything you do, but you should not criticize and belittle yourself if your job isn't perfect. If you've done your best, that's all you can possibly be expected to do.

15. Learn to control your competitive nature. The highway is a good place to practice this: When you see a car trying to edge in from a side road, pause long enough to let it in the stream of traffic instead of hitting the accelerator until you pass him and keep him off the road. Contribute to a discussion without trying to create an argument and win it. Learn to take it easy; chances are, nobody else even views the situation as a competition, anyway.

16. Get enough sleep. This is critical: Sleep helps your body recover from stress by allowing it time to heal and slow down.

17. Learn to concentrate on a task or job while you are doing it. Fight the tendency to let your mind wander to some other problem or task until you have finished the one you are working on.

18. Learn how to say no to things that you don't want to do. Too many people feel guilty about saying no, but you are the master of your own self and you have the freedom to choose how you spend your time and energies. Don't get involved in something you don't really want to do just because you couldn't say no.

19. Periodically get up from your work and stretch. If you need to go some-where else in the building, take the stairs. If you need to go to an appointment a few blocks away, walk—don't drive. Walk briskly around the office or building periodically during the day. If you are able to take a break, go outside and get some fresh air, even if it's winter.

20. Try some instant relaxers whenever you feel stress coming on: Bend at the waist, letting your arms dangle, and sway slowly from side to side. Drop your chin to your chest and rotate your head slowly in a complete circle. Tilt your head several times to each side in a bouncing motion. Massage your neck (or, better yet, have someone else rub your neck and shoulders). Lie down with your feet elevated for fifteen minutes.

21. Learn—and practice—yoga or some other meditation form.

22. Eat the proper kinds of foods in the proper amounts. People under stress have greater nutritional needs than people who are not prone to stress. It is critical that you get enough protein, vitamins, and minerals to repair the tissues that have been damaged as a result of stress. Avoid starchy, sugary food and empty junk food calories; eat a well-balanced diet that includes meat, dairy foods, fresh fruits, and fresh vegetables as well as whole grains found in breads and cereals. Keep your weight down, too. Excess weight places extra strain on the same body organs and functions that stress does—and it might be the straw that breaks *your* back.

23. Realize and appreciate your own value as a human being with potential and talent.

24. Allow yourself to express your emotions freely within the bounds of appropriateness. If you are saddened by the death of a close friend, let yourself cry. If someone makes you angry, let yourself express your anger reasonably. Letting yourself express your emotion helps you to deal with it better.

25. If you have difficulty dealing with someone that you are forced to interact with on a daily or regular basis (such as a close colleague), approach the person in a calm and rational manner and let him or her know what it is that upsets you. Don't use language such as *"You always* chew your pencils" or *"You never* empty the garbage can by the desk.'' Instead, say something like ''*I* have a hard time concentrating when you chew your pencil'' or ''It's hard for *me* to remember to empty the garbage can next to the desk every day; can we split the job and each take two days a week?'' Using an approach such as this will help you get your problem out in the open without creating an unpleasant, threatening situation for you or the other person.

26. Hurrying is a learned behavior; it can be changed. If you have the tendency to hurry, think about it. Slow down when you can. Plan far enough ahead so that you aren't always in a rush. Make allowances for activities that are scheduled, and realistically assess what you can accomplish before that time. Remember: You don't *have* to hurry. Drive to the grocery store well within the speed limit; wheel the cart around the store at a leisurely pace. Enjoy a walk to class or work; leave home in enough time to get there with a walk, not a run.

27. Love people around you. Start with your family; tell them you love them. Try it on your roommate, a friend. Try loving people and using things instead of the other way around.

28. Use music to help calm yourself down. The music should be quiet, soothing, and instrumental; listening lying down, with your eyes closed. Fall asleep if you can; use the time to take a short nap.

29. Take active steps to manage your environment; pinpoint the things in your everyday surroundings that cause you stress and eliminate or change as many of them as you can. If the telephone is a constant bother while you are trying to concentrate, temporarily unplug it. If your appointment book is a source of stress, ask your secretary to take care of it and simply to remind you of your obligations.

30. Let people know what they can expect of you and how much time you are willing to give them. This goes back to the ability to say no. If people ask you to serve on a committee, let them first know exactly how much time you are willing to devote to your committee work. Tell them firmly that is all the time you can spend; tell them that if the committee assignment will require more time than you have specified, you will not serve on the committee. And watch out: Someone may try to urge you into spending excess time later, after you have agreed to serve. Stick to your guns. You made yourself clear ahead of time, and you deserve to be respected.

31. Practice eating more slowly. Put your fork down in between bites; take a sip of water frequently. Eating is a basic habit, and if you're able to slow it down, you can slow down other things, too.

32. Try doing everything more slowly once you have mastered the skill of eating slowly. Walk more slowly; talk more slowly. Watch yourself as you talk: Are your gestures wild and rapid?

33. Set your own guidelines and standards for behavior. Quit worrying about what everyone else thinks; if you're happy, that's what is important.

34. Try to be positive in your outlook. It's easy to be critical and to find the negative in people and things. For a week try to find the positive instead. Think about that house you pass every day on the way to work—you know, the one that really gets under your skin. Try noticing how well manicured the yard is and how nicely trimmed the shrubs along the front windows are instead of the fact that someone painted the trim a lime green. Once you get into the habit of looking for the positive, you'll find that your whole outlook—and your entire frame of mind—changes for the better. You'll be less upset by things. After all, you can't change that awful lime green trim; you might as well learn to live with it.

35. Everyone makes mistakes. Try using yours to your advantage. Instead of dwelling on some bad experience, building up a pressure cooker of guilt and shame, turn the experience around and decide what positive things you can learn from it. Choose something that's bothered you for a long time—maybe the time you were indifferent toward a college roommate, say, and his loneliness caused him to leave school. Quit thinking of the experience only in terms of what you did wrong and how you are to blame. Look at it in terms of what you learned: Now you have the opportunity of being a caring, responsible friend for those who need someone to talk to or someone to turn to for friendship. You can recognize those needs, and many people aren't able to.

36. Treat those around you with respect. It's easy to get suspicious and paranoid about people who are causing you stress. Instead of lashing out with hostility, try treating them with courtesy and respect. They'll probably return the favor, and you may find that they don't cause you that much stress, after all.

37. Do what you can to improve relationships that are important to you. It might be a romantic partner, a sister who is attending the same university you are, the grandmother with whom you are living. An important and major source of stress stems from personal relationships; do what you can to make sure yours are working as well as they can.

38. Remember that there are always options and alternatives. All of us make plans, and all of us are disappointed when our plans do not materialize or when things do not go as we would wish them to. It is *not* the end of the world—or even a major crisis—if something doesn't work out for you. Remember: There are *always* options. Take a deep breath, sit down, and figure out a different way of accomplishing your goal or dream. You are in command if you take the time and intelligence to be in command.

39. Get in touch with your needs. Each of us is an individual, and each of us has unique needs. We all have the basic ones—the need for security, for nourishment, for sleep, for warmth—but you probably have one or two (and probably many more) that are unique. Take the time to know yourself well, and figure out what your own needs are. Maybe you need to get outside into the sunshine every day; maybe you need to render service to someone else every day in order to feel fulfilled; maybe you need to develop a closer relationship with your professors in order to grasp the course material. Once you've found out what your needs are, set about working on ways to fulfill them. If your own unique needs go unmet—even if you're not sure what they are—you will feel frustrated and unhappy, often without knowing why.

The most important keys to managing stress are to involve yourself in activities you enjoy and to eliminate sources of stress from your life. If your mother wants you to be a veterinarian but you want to be an accountant, choose a college curriculum that will allow you to fulfill your own goal and do the thing that makes you happiest. If you decide to develop a regular program of exercise, choose activities that are fun for you: jumping rope when it's blizzardy outside, playing tennis when it's warm. When you look for a job, find something that you enjoy doing. One person might love organizing files while another might enjoy sitting at a receptionist desk. If you experience stress when you are forced to interact with strangers, don't accept a job sitting at a receptionist desk, no matter how desperate you are for the money. Hold out for something that will allow you to relax—maybe the files are just for you.

In other words, make good choices for *you.* Don't do something because it's expected or because everyone else is doing it. Don't buy season tickets to the football games if football bores you; consider tickets to the symphony instead or spend your Saturday afternoons building a car for your younger brother to race in the Soap Box Derby.

Take control. Take it easy. And, above all, have fun. Once you have learned to value yourself as a person, you will find it easy to protect yourself from the ravages of diseases caused by needless stress.

SELF-EVALUATION TEST
PART I

Check which events have happened to you in the past twelve months (one year) and record the score indicated. Do not count an event twice. For example, if your job has changed, do not check both "Change to a different line of work" and "Change in responsibilities at work;" instead, select which event most closely describes the change you made and score that.

Event Value	Event	Your Score
100	Death of spouse	
73	Divorce	
65	Marital separation	
63	Jail term	
63	Death of close family member	

Event Value	Event	Your Score
53	Personal injury or illness	
50	Marriage	
47	Fired from job	
45	Marital reconciliation	
45	Retirement	
44	Change in health of family member	
40	Pregnancy	
39	Sexual difficulties	
39	Gain of new family member	
39	Business readjustment	
38	Change in financial state	
37	Death of a close friend	
36	Change to a different line of work	
35	Change in number of arguments with spouse	
31	Mortgage over $10,000	
30	Foreclosure of mortgage or loan	
29	Change in responsibilities at work	
29	Son or daughter leaving home	
29	Trouble with in-laws	
28	Outstanding personal achievement	
26	Spouse begins or stops work	
26	Begin or end school	
25	Change in living conditions	
24	Revision of personal habits	
23	Trouble with boss	
20	Change in work hours or conditions	
20	Change in residence	
20	Change in schools	
19	Change in recreation	
19	Change in church activities	
18	Change in social activities	
17	Mortgage or loan less than $10,000	
16	Change in sleeping habits	
15	Change in number of family get-togethers	
15	Change in eating habits	
13	Vacation	
12	Christmas	
11	Minor violations of the law	

(Reprinted with permission of Pergamon Press, Inc., and Thomas H. Holmes.)

SCORING

If your score is 300 or more, you have an 80-percent chance of developing a serious stress-related illness within the next two years. Similar severe illnesses will be suffered by 53 percent of those whose scores were 250–300, and by 33 percent of those whose scores were 150–200. (*Stress-related illness* refers to any illness that can be affected by stress; such illnesses include asthma, cancer, heart failure, and many other diseases and illnesses. Remember that an estimated 80 percent of people who see doctors do so because of stress-related illnesses; many doctors now believe that *all* illness is caused, at least in part, by stress.)

PART II:
DETERMINING YOUR RISK

Circle the characteristics that apply to you:

Mental	Physical
Feeling of unease	Overweight
Irritability	High blood pressure
Boredom with life	Lack of appetite
Feeling of inability to cope	Desire to eat when problems arise
Anxiety about money	Frequent heartburn
Morbid fear of disease	Chronic diarrhea
Morbid fear of cancer	Chronic constipation
Fear of death (your own and others')	Inability to sleep
Sense of suppressed anger	Constant fatigue
Inability to express emotion	Frequent headaches
Inability to have a good laugh	Need for medication every day
Feeling of family rejection	Muscle spasms
Feeling of failure as parent	Feeling of fullness without eating
Dread of weekends	Unexplained shortness of breath
Reluctance to take a vacation	Fainting attacks
Inability to discuss problems	Nausea
Inability to concentrate	Inability to cry
Inability to finish a job	Tendency to burst into tears at
Terror of heights	slight provocation
Terror of enclosed spaces	Frigidity
Fear of thunderstorms	Impotence
	Fear of intercourse
	Excess nervous energy
	Inability to sit still
	Inability to relax physically

SCORING
You have a high risk of developing stress-related problems if you circled more than two of the physical signs, more than four of the mental signs, or a total of four of the mental and physical signs.

REFERENCES

[1]Curriculum Concepts, Inc., *Stress!* (Chicago, Ill.: American Hospital Association, 1977), p. 4.

[2]Donald B. Ardell, *High Level Wellness* (Emmaus, Pa.: Rodale Press, 1977), p. 134; also cited in Hans Selye, *Stress Without Distress* (New York: J. B. Lippincott Company, 1974), p. 111.

[3]Matthew J. Culligan and Keith Sedlacek, *How to Kill Stress Before It Kills You* (New York: Grosset & Dunlap, Inc., 1976), p. 36.

[4]*Feel Younger—Live Longer* (New York: Rand McNally & Company, 1976), p. 74.

[5]Donald M. Vickery, *LifePlan for Your Health* (Reading, Mass.: Addison-Wesley Publishing Co., Inc., 1978), pp. 184–85.

[6]Tom Hirsh, "Stress," *National Safety News,* January 1979, p. 38.

[7]Ibid., pp. 34–35, 36, 38.

[8]Ibid., p. 34.

[9]Curriculum Concepts, *Stress!,* p. 12; *Feel Younger—Live Longer,* pp. 82–83; Richard M. Suinn, "How to Break the Vicious Cycle of Stress," *Psychology Today,* December 1976, pp. 59–60.

[10]Thomas H. Holmes and Minoru Masuda, "Psychosomatic Syndrome," *Psychology Today,* April 1972, pp. 23–24.

[11]Ibid.

[12]Ibid.

[13]Claude A. Frazier, "The Anxious Mind and Disease," *Nursing Care,* January 1977, p. 17.

[14]W. P. Wilson and B. S. Nashold, "Pain and Emotion," *Postgraduate Medicine,* May 1970, p. 184.

[15]A. Lynn Cope, "Pain: Its Psychological Aspects," *Journal of Practical Nursing,* January 1977, p. 30.

[16]Ibid., p. 31.

[17]Joel E. Dimsdale, "Emotional Causes of Sudden Death," *American Journal of Psychiatry*, 134, no. 12 (December 1977), 1361.

[18]J. G. Bruhn, A. Paredes, and C. A. Adsett, "Psychological Predictors of Sudden Death in Myocardial Infarction," *Journal of Psychosomatic Research*, 18 (1974), 187–91.

HEART
DISEASE
THE NUMBER-ONE KILLER

"Pass the salt, please." . . . *"No, I'm too tired this morning—let's* drive *over to campus."* . . . *"I piled on twenty pounds last year!"* . . . *"I tried to cut down on my smoking once, but sales conferences make me so nervous."*

Heart disease is the number-one killer in the United States today; more than a million people die from it each year, and over 29 million of us are afflicted with some form of it.[1]

And ironically, you can do more to prevent your chances of being affected by heart disease than you can do to combat any other major cause of death.

By the way, heart disease isn't just a disease of the middle-aged executive with gray hair sprinkled around his temples and a paunch tucked under his belt. It isn't just a disease of white-haired old ladies whose gnarled hands grip the edges of wheelchairs. Scan the obituaries in your local paper some morning: Heart disease is claiming its victims from college campuses; the grim black-and-white faces looking back at you are those of mothers, executives, and other people just like you.

But you don't have to be there in those narrow columns if you don't want to be. Heart disease, for the most part, is preventable. All it takes is a basic understanding of how your heart works, what factors affect your heart's performance, what things you do that present a risk for your heart, and how you can overcome those risks.

HOW YOUR HEART WORKS

Your heart, your body's pump, begins working before you are even born; if you are lucky, it will continue to pump blood throughout your body nonstop for eighty or ninety years. If for some reason it stops pumping for longer than four minutes, you will die.[2]

The heart's job isn't an easy one. While you are resting, it pumps 10 pints of blood every minute; it can increase this performance by five times—pumping up to 6.25 gallons every minute—for brief periods of time while you are exercising heavily. During a single day—twenty-four hours—it pumps 3,000–5,000 gallons of blood. That's 1.4 million gallons every year, or a whopping 100 million gallons during an eighty-year lifetime—enough to fill the tanks of over 2,000 four-engine Boeing 747 airplanes!

How—and why—does this pumping take place?

The reason your heart pumps, of course, is to circulate blood throughout your body to all of the organs and cells that make up the complex network of systems that digest your food, do your thinking, run across a football field, and reproduce children. Blood that leaves the heart is filled with life-giving nutrients, oxygen, water, and minerals that are needed by your cells. The blood courses through arteries that lead finally to microscopic capillaries that nourish even the smallest cells. On its way back to the heart the blood is laden with waste products—excess water, carbon dioxide, and metabolic by-products. On its journey through the kidneys and lungs the blood is purified and restocked with nutrients, ready to be sent out again by the heart to the trillions of cells that make up your body.

The vast network of blood vessels that carry blood from the heart to each microscopic cell would stretch 60,000 miles if they were lined up end to end: almost two and a half times around the earth at the equator. Yet your miraculous heart moves your blood through this complex network and back to itself—all in approximately ten seconds.

Sometimes other things are circulated by the heart in the blood: Hormones, drugs, and glandular secretions often join the blood on its journey as it wends its way throughout your body.

How does the heart work?

The heart is actually a double pump consisting of four chambers. One pumping station, involving two of the heart's chambers, is located on the left; the other pumping station, involving the heart's other two chambers, is located on the right. The two sides are separated, but they pump at the same time. The chambers on the top are called *atria*, and they are the blood-receiving chambers; the blood-pumping chambers on the bottom are called the *ventricles*.

Oxygen-poor blood laden with waste products enters the heart through a huge vein, the superior vena cava, which dumps the blood into the right atrium;

the blood passes from the right atrium through the tricuspid valve into the right ventricle, where it is pumped through another valve and into the pulmonary artery, which carries the blood to the lungs.

As the blood circulates through the lungs, the carbon dioxide and other metabolic by-products are filtered out, and the blood is impregnated with freshly inhaled oxygen. It then returns to the heart via the pulmonary vein.

From the pulmonary vein the freshly oxygenated blood is pumped into the left atrium, through the mitral valve and left ventricle and into the aorta, the major artery that starts the blood on its journey through the body.

From the aorta the blood passes into smaller arteries, which then carry it to all the body organs and tissues. Once it reaches the organs and tissues, it passes into the arterioles, the smallest arterial branches, and finally into capillaries, dense networks of tiny, thin-walled blood vessels that reach individual cell clusters. Because the walls of the capillaries are so thin, exchange of elements is easy: The oxygen and other nutrients from the blood pass into the cell, and the blood absorbs carbon dioxide and other metabolic by-products from the cell.

The blood then starts its journey back to the heart—from the capillaries to the venules (the smallest veins), from the venules to the veins, and finally to the superior vena cava, where the blood is dumped again into the right atrium and the process begins all over again.

Remember: It took only ten seconds for that entire journey, start to finish.

DIAGNOSING HEART DISEASE

Medical researchers have refined a number of tests and diagnostic tools that enable them to determine the presence—and degree of involvement—of heart disease.* If you or your doctor suspect that you might have some type of heart disease, you may be given one or more of the following tests:

BLOOD TEST

By drawing a sample of your blood and examining it under a microscope, doctors can determine the amount of certain elements in your blood. One important determinant of heart disease is the amount of fats lipids—particularly triglycerides and cholesterol—in the blood; the only way to determine that level is to examine a sample of blood.

A blood test may also reveal to your doctor the presence of abnormal blood sugar, a sign indicating possible diabetes (another major cause of heart disease).

*This section adapted from John Ross, Jr., and Robert A. O'Rourke, *Understanding the Heart and Its Diseases* (New York: McGraw-Hill Book Company, 1976), pp. 25–42.

ELECTROCARDIOGRAM

Commonly referred to as an ECG or EKG, the electrocardiogram gives a graphic representation of the electrical activity of the heart; sensitive equipment placed on the skin surface of your chest traces electrical impulses onto graph paper, where they can be read and interpreted by specialists. An EKG is almost always taken while the patient is lying down at rest.

An EKG can reveal irregularities in the heart rhythm and can disclose which portion of the heart muscle sustained injury as a result of a heart attack or other heart disorder.

CHEST X RAY

Two specific disorders—enlargement of the heart and impairment of the circulatory system in the lungs—can be diagnosed by chest X ray. To be completely effective, the X ray should reveal the entire chest structure, including the heart, the ribs, the lungs, the blood vessels, and the area immediately surrounding them.

EXERCISE ELECTROCARDIOGRAM

Designed to determine how much stress the heart can withstand, an exercise electrocardiogram is taken while the patient is exercising; the same kind of tracing equipment and graph paper is used as in the electrocardiogram taken at rest. Because it is designed to diagnose certain disorders that only affect the heart when it is under stress, it is important that the person undergoing the exercise electrocardiogram elevate his or her heartbeat to a rate that approximates stress (or heavy exercise).

Most often the exercise electrocardiogram is taken while the patient walks or runs on a treadmill, pedals on a stationary bicycle, or walks up and down a short flight of stairs. Because a damaged heart may act up during an exercise electrocardiogram, such a test is performed in a hospital while a team of doctors stands by.

FLUOROSCOPE

A fluoroscope is similar to an X ray because it allows the doctor to view the internal organs of the chest by means of small doses of radiation. But whereas an X ray presents a still picture, a fluoroscope allows the doctor to watch the heart in motion. Equipment is attached to the patient's chest wall, and the doctor views the "shadows" on a monitoring television screen.

Fluoroscopy is used in diagnosing calcification (hardening of the valves and vessels of the heart), irregularities in heart function, and irregularities in heart chamber size.

Fluoroscopy is often used in combination with other tests.

PHONOCARDIOLOGY

By means of a series of microphones that are placed on the chest wall and connected to sensitive recording devices, phonocardiology records even the most minute heart sounds.

The doctor can either listen to the sounds as they are emitted, or the equipment can be attached to an oscilloscope, which allows the sound patterns to be either photographed or traced on graph paper.

ECHOCARDIOGRAPHY

Similar in technique to sonar—which is used at sea to determine depth and to locate underwater objects—echocardiography can reveal the size of the heart chambers and great vessels, the motion of the heart valves, and the shape of the heart chambers and vessels.

To record these images, a small device is placed on the skin surface of the chest; pulses of sound are then transmitted into the chest (the sound is ultrasound, and cannot be detected by human ears). The echoes returning from the surfaces of the heart are electronically recorded and plotted on graph paper.

CARDIAC CATHETER

A thin, flexible tube made of material to which blood will not adhere (such as woven plastic) is threaded to the heart through a vein or artery (usually of the arm or leg). A cardiac catheter makes it possible to draw blood samples from the heart itself and to measure blood pressure in the individual heart chambers, across the heart valves, or across the great vessels.

Because the cardiac catheter procedure requires hospitalization and careful follow-up observation (and because it requires general anesthesia), it is usually performed over a period of several days.

DISEASES
OF THE HEART

Seven major diseases affect the heart and its system: hypertension (high blood pressure), heart attack, congestive heart failure, stroke, atherosclerosis, arteriosclerosis, rheumatic heart disease, and congenital heart disease.

HIGH BLOOD PRESSURE

Without pressure the blood couldn't circulate through the body; the pressure necessary to circulate the blood is created by the contractions of the heart and by the resistance of the arterial walls. Every time the heart beats, the pressure goes up and down within a limited range. In some cases, it goes up and stays up—a condition known as high blood pressure (hypertension).

One in every six adults in the United States has high blood pressure.[3] It's a major killer, leading to congestive heart failure, stroke, and kidney failure. And it's a mysterious, silent killer; 90 percent of those who have high blood pressure have it for reasons that remain unknown, and most of them manifest no symptoms.[4] At present, there is no cure, only methods of control and prevention.

MEASURING BLOOD PRESSURE

You've probably had a test for blood pressure. An inflatable rubber cuff (called a sphygmomanometer) is wrapped around the upper arm; a sufficient amount of air to cut off the circulation is pumped into the cuff.

As the air is gradually let out of the cuff, the technician listens with a stethoscope as the first blood rushes through the artery, noting the pressure on the gauge as he or she hears the first sound of rushing blood. Pressure at that point is called *systolic,* the amount of pressure exerted when the heart contracts. A systolic pressure of about 120 is considered normal (if you are older than forty-five, a slightly higher reading is still considered normal).[5]

The technician continues to release air from the cuff until the sounds of the blood become muffled or disappear; the technician again checks the gauge. This number is a measurement of the *diastolic* pressure, the lowest level of pressure exerted, between beats, when the heart is at rest. A diastolic pressure of about 80 is considered normal (again, normal is slightly higher for these over forty-five).[6]

From the two numbers noted at your systolic and diastolic pressures, you get your blood pressure: 120/80 if your systolic pressure is 120 and your diastolic pressure is 80.

At any age a systolic pressure of 160 or more and a diastolic pressure of 95 or more is considered dangerous.[7]

CAUSES

Researchers are unsure as to the exact causes of high blood pressure, but we are aware of some contributing factors that seem to lead to its development:

Heredity. Hypertension often runs in families;[8] this may be due either to strict genetic factors or to the fact that family members usually have the same general life-style—and life-style has been shown to be a leading factor in the development of high blood pressure.

Race. Black people are more likely to develop high blood pressure; hypertension is the major disease among America's black population and is the major factor in their shorter life expectancy.[9]

Emotional tension and stress. Blood pressure naturally goes up during periods of emotional crisis because the body is preparing itself for an emergency. Some people, however, react to life as if it were a series of emergencies, and their bodies never have a chance to calm down and return to normal. Especially prone are individuals with a type-A personality, as discussed in the last chapter. Stress is considered to be one of the leading factors in development of high blood pressure.[10]

Smoking. Nicotine is known to raise blood pressure chemically; heavy cigarette smoking is known to be a factor in the development of hypertension.[11]

Body chemistry. For some unknown reason, some people secrete into the bloodstream chemicals that cause high blood pressure; these secretions generally originate in the kidneys or the adrenal glands.[12]

Diet high in fats and salt. Fats and salt act together chemically, to accelerate the development of atherosclerosis, which in turn leads to heart attacks, stroke, and the development of high blood pressure.[13] According to some researchers, too much salt ingested at an early age (especially in baby food) can cause a predisposition toward high blood pressure later in life. Hypertension occurs four times as often in Japan as in the United States, possibly due to the fact that the Japanese eat an average of seven teaspoons of salt a day.[14]

Kidney defects. A common contributing factor to high blood pressure is an obstruction of the blood flow to the kidneys.[15]

Adrenal cortex defects. Defects of the adrenal cortex cause it to secrete aldosterone (or a similar hormone), which causes the body to retain sodium, resulting in the same condition as would occur if you ate too much salt. Most adrenal cortex defects are caused by small tumors on the adrenal gland.[16]

Diseases of the pituitary, thyroid, or parathyroid glands.[17]

Toxemia.[18]

Blood and blood vessel defects (generally due to birth defects).[19]

Obesity.[20]

SYMPTOMS

Unfortunately, hypertension rarely exhibits any symptoms at all—as mentioned earlier, 90 percent of those who have high blood pressure are unaware that anything at all is wrong.* There is usually no pain.

If symptoms do occur, they generally include nagging headaches in the back of the head and upper part of the neck; dizziness; shortness of breath; excessive flushing of the face; fatigue; and insomnia.

Remember, most cases of high blood pressure don't manifest any pain or symptoms. It would be foolish to wait for symptoms to develop; by the time something *did* show up, it would probably be too late for effective treatment. The best way to detect high blood pressure is to have your blood pressure measured during a regular physical examination.

Treatment for high blood pressure generally consists of drug programs aimed at reducing the blood pressure. High blood pressure can be controlled, but it cannot be cured.

WHAT CAN YOU DO?

There are things that you can do now to protect yourself against developing high blood pressure. Consider the following:

Cut down on salt. This is probably one of the most important ways you can fight the development of high blood pressure. We need about 230 milligrams of sodium (found in ordinary table salt) every day—but some estimates cite that Americans consume about *twenty times* that amount. Consider these seemingly harmless foods: one serving of corn flakes contains 260 milligrams; a serving of jello has 404 milligrams; one slice of American cheese contains 238 milligrams; a serving of canned peas, 349 milligrams; canned tomato juice, 292 milligrams; a dill pickel, a whopping 1137 milligrams; and a serving of instant beef broth, 818 milligrams. Other culprits include things like bacon, bologna, potato chips, bottled salad dressing, tuna fish, catsup, peanut butter, and TV dinners.[21]

Because we get so much salt already in the foods we eat, watch your intake of table salt. Most of us pick up the salt shaker out of habit, anyway; how many times do you taste your food before you salt it?

Stop smoking.

Lose weight if you need to. Every pound of fat that you add to your body must be nourished by blood vessels; every pound of fat, then, places an added burden on the heart. If you're overweight for your height and frame, your heart is

*This section adapted from Theodore Irwin, *Watch Your Blood Pressure*, rev. ed. (Bethesda, Md.: U.S. Department of Health, Education and Welfare, National Institutes of Health, Public Affairs Commission, 1976), pp. 7–8.

forced to pump more blood through a larger network of blood vessels, and the added work is a major cause of high blood pressure.

Exercise. Before you embark on any program of exercise, you should check with your doctor; if you're really out of shape, you should have a physical exam first. Why? If you dive in too quickly and try to do too much too soon, you could end up overworking your heart and creating worse problems than you're trying to prevent. Mild exercise, such as walking or light jogging, can be beneficial in lowering high blood pressure; rigorous exercise, however, can be dangerous. If you're in the clear and the doctor gives you the go-ahead, work out an exercise program that gives you some kind of physical activity every day and some kind of vigorous exercise at least once a week.[22]

Calm down. Stress is a highly suspicious culprit in the cause of high blood pressure—and people who are under a great deal of stress need to take steps to relieve it.[23] Study the previous chapter; it lists a number of good suggestions that might help you in overcoming problems with stress, especially if you are a type-A personality.

Check with your doctor before you use birth control pills. Although scientific proof is not conclusive, we do have evidence that *some* people may react in such a way to *some* kinds of oral contraceptives as to develop high blood pressure.[24] Your doctor can help monitor your reactions to birth control pills and can advise you about which kinds are the safest for you to use.

HEART ATTACK

Over half the people who die from heart disease die from heart attack; almost 700,000 Americans each year succumb to heart attacks. Many more suffer attacks each year and live.[25]

Heart attack refers to a situation when an artery of the heart becomes blocked (either by fatty deposits, such as in atherosclerosis, or by a blood clot, such as in a stroke) and impairs the flow of blood to the heart muscle and tissue. When an artery becomes obstructed, the heart muscle tissue beyond that artery dies; death of heart tissue is referred to as *myocardial infarction.* As a result of the myocardial infarction, the heart muscle may suddenly quiver, a condition referred to as *ventricular fibrillation.* Ventricular fibrillation, unless corrected immediately (within seconds), leads to death. A myocardial infarction may or may not cause death, depending on the amount of tissue that dies.[26]

CAUSES

As mentioned before, a heart attack results when an artery of the heart is blocked—either by a fatty deposit or by a blood clot.

Heart attacks seem to be sudden, but they're not: life-style patterns and ways of living throughout an entire lifetime affect the arteries of the heart.[27] By learning the risk factors and the early warning signs, you can take measures to avert heart attack before it ever strikes.

Some factors that contribute to heart attack include

- Overweight, especially extreme overweight (thirty or more pounds exceeding ideal weight for height and frame)
- High blood pressure
- Smoking
- Lack of exercise and general sedentary life-style (at particular risk are those with sedentary jobs who do not have a regular program of exercise)
- Diabetes (including family history of diabetes)
- Family history of heart attack among immediate family members (parents, brothers, sisters)
- High blood cholesterol level (generally over 225 mg.)
- Stress
- Previous heart problems (such as a murmur or extra heart beats)

WARNING SIGNS

Pain, in one form or another, almost always accompanies heart attack. Some heart attacks will produce pain that is only a mild ache; others will be accompanied by pain of almost unbearable intensity. Pain can be in any of the following areas: localized under the breastbone; large area of the midchest, sometimes involving entire upper chest; midchest, radiating to the neck and lower jaw; midchest, radiating to the inside arms (the left arm and shoulder is more commonly involved than the right); the upper abdomen (often mistaken for indigestion); the midchest or large area of the chest, neck, jaw, and inside of arms; lower center neck, radiating to both sides of the upper neck and along the jaw from ear to ear; the inside of right arm from armpit to just below elbow, and inside of left arm from armpit to waist (may also involve left shoulder); and back, between shoulder blades.[28]

Besides pain, early warning signs of heart attack include difficulty in breathing, heart palpitations, nausea, vomiting, cold sweats, paleness, weakness, and a sense of anxiety or impending doom.[29]

DISTINGUISHING CHEST PAIN

How can you tell if the pain in your chest is a warning of heart attack and not some other problem (such as indigestion, heartburn, or bursitis)?

50

The heart is in the center of the chest, *not* on the left side. The pain is rarely sharp or jabbing: Pain in the heart is a result of oxygen supply being cut off, and pain from heart attack is more often a feeling of pressure, fullness, squeezing, or aching. It can come and go, often over a period of weeks or months. Don't be fooled if the pain goes away; your heart is trying to warn you that danger is just around the corner.

If you have a pain in your chest, try lifting your arms above your head. If the pain is due to arthritis, bursitis, or muscle strain, movement of the arms as you lift them over your head will make the pain get temporarily worse. There will be no change in the pain due to heart attack.

If the pain is in your neck, turn your head to either side and then bend your head forward. If you have a stiff neck due to muscle tension or strain, swollen glands, arthritis, or a toothache, the pain will intensify when you move your head and neck. Heart attack pain will not respond to movement.

Cough and breathe deeply. If your pain is due to a broken rib, respiratory infection, hiatal hernia, pinched nerve, arthritis, ulcer, gallbladder problem, overexertion, or malnourishment, the pain will worsen as you cough or breathe deeply. In some cases movement may ease the pain. Heart attack pain will neither worsen nor ease up from movement.

In addition to feeling a squeezing, aching, or pressing pain, you may feel a sense of impending doom or strong emotion.

Pain in the left chest wall, centering on the left nipple, is almost never a sign of heart attack. Pain suffered on the left side of the chest may be either dull and aching or sharp and jabbing; it is a common occurrence among victims of stress and is often mistaken for heart attack.

If you suspect that you may be suffering from a heart attack, get to a hospital immediately. It is not safe to drive yourself; have a friend or family member take you if someone is available to drive you immediately; call an ambulance or a paramedic team if someone cannot drive you to the hospital. If you can, call your doctor before you leave for the hospital so that he or she can meet you there and can make arrangements to provide for your care once you reach the hospital.

Once you reach the hospital, insist on immediate care.

If you have access to nitroglycerin tablets, put one under your tongue as soon as you determine that you may be having a heart attack; it will ease your distress within a few minutes. (This is one of the rare instances when self-medication is justified.)

Go to the nearest hospital. It's a smart idea to find out ahead of time where the nearest hospital is, what facilities it has, where the emergency room entrance is, and how you can reach the hospital the fastest. Finding out this information should be a matter of routine each time you settle in a new community. The next time you see your doctor, find out where you should go in the hospital to get the quickest care, regardless of the complaint or injury.

PREVENTING HEART ATTACK

There are a number of things you can do to prevent heart attack or to reduce your risk of having a heart attack.

Be alert for the signs of heart attack. Your heart may warn you for weeks or months before the actual attack occurs, or you may suffer a minor heart attack without really being disabled. Many people suffer "little" heart attacks and don't heed the signs that are manifest—and once you have had a heart attack, you are much more prone to have others. (People who recover from one heart attack—be it major or minor in nature—are five times more likely to die within the next five years from a heart attack than are people who have no history of heart attack.)

Reduce your weight to the normal level for your height and frame. Overweight is one of the most common and most far-reaching factors leading to heart attack, particularly since it contributes to atherosclerosis and high blood pressure, two of the major causes of heart attack.

Develop an exercise program that involves some kind of activity every day and some kind of vigorous exercise at least once a week. If you are out of shape or have been sedentary for quite a while, check with a doctor before you undergo any kind of exercise program—you should probably be given a stress test to measure how much exercise your heart can tolerate.

Reduce the amount of cholesterol in your diet. Also restrict the amount of fat you consume. *Some* fat is needed, so don't make the mistake of eliminating it completely. Recent research suggests that highly saturated fats contribute to the formation of low-density lipoproteins, which are more of a factor in creating fatty deposits on the artery walls than high-density lipoproteins. To help increase the proportion of the desirable high-density lipoproteins (HDL), you should exercise vigorously, reduce your intake of saturated fats, and eat plenty of fruits and vegetables.

If you have high blood pressure, check with your doctor for treatment. Make sure that you follow his therapy program precisely so that the hypertension stays under control.

Quit smoking.

If you have diabetes, check with your doctor and stick to a program that will help keep the disease in check.

Eliminate stress and tension from your life as much as possible. Learn to identify which situations cause you excessive stress, and take steps to avoid them or to compensate for them. The chapter on stress offers valuable suggestions for learning to control stress.

WHAT IF YOU'VE HAD A HEART ATTACK?

If you've already had a heart attack, you will need to adopt certain dietary, exercise, and life-style restrictions to protect yourself from suffering another heart attack. Generally, your doctor will be able to instruct you as to prevention techniques, but the following are pretty universal:

Follow a diet low in carbohydrates. Low-carbohydrate diet can help you eliminate fluids that you might otherwise retain.

Make sure that you get a well-balanced diet that includes food rich in minerals and vitamins. Some research indicates that such trace elements as zinc, copper, manganese, and selenium help prevent a second heart attack and help reduce chest pain that lingers after a first heart attack.

Limit consumption of alcohol. Instead of stimulating the heart, as is so often believed, alcohol works as a depressant to slow down the heart. Limit yourself to one drink each day; for two hours after you do drink, avoid any strenuous activity that might trigger a heart attack.

Exercise regularly. Don't lift heavy weights, shovel snow, push heavy objects (like pianos or cars), or do upper arm exercises or isometric exercises. You *can* safely jog, walk, run, bike, dance, swim, play volleyball, and do calisthenics if you build up your activity gradually and if you have your doctor's approval.

CONGESTIVE HEART FAILURE

Congestive heart failure is *not* a heart attack—but a heart attack is one of the things that can cause congestive heart failure.

Congestive heart failure results when the heart muscle has been damaged by heart attack, rheumatic fever, atherosclerosis, high blood pressure, or birth defects. As a result of the damage to the tissue, the heart's pumping capacity is reduced well below normal. The result? Fluids begin to accummulate in the extremities and in the lungs.[30]

SYMPTOMS

Symptoms of congestive heart failure include fatigue; shortness of breath, first when you exert yourself, later when you are resting; difficulty in breathing at night, including wheezing; swelling of the legs, ankles, and feet, with difficulty getting shoes on or off or the necessity of changing to a larger shoe size; swelling of the hands and fingers, with difficulty in removing rings; puffiness of the face; a sudden weight gain with no change in diet; a feeling of being waterlogged or bloated; and an accumulation of fluid in the lungs.[31]

Treatment regimes include limiting salt intake, a program of weight loss, and carefully monitored exercise designed to avoid putting stress on the heart. Drug therapy is usually undertaken to help the body rid itself of excess fluids and to increase the pumping action of the heart.[32]

PREVENTION

The key to prevention of congestive heart failure is to prevent damage to the heart muscle—in other words, take measures to prevent high blood pressure, heart attack, and atherosclerosis; get prompt treatment for rheumatic fever; and follow a therapeutic program to help deal with congenital heart disease.

STROKE

Over 200,000 people die from strokes in the United States each year; approximately 300,000 suffer strokes and survive. Over 21 million people in this country have high blood pressure, which is the leading cause of stroke.[33]

WHAT IS STROKE?

A stroke is an accident involving a blood vessel—most of the time it involves a blood vessel in the brain. For some reason the blood supply is cut off to the brain because the artery can no longer carry the blood normally. There are five reasons why damage occurs to the arteries:[34]

Hemorrhage. Due to high blood pressure or some forms of disease (including infection of the arteries), a wall of the artery may burst, causing blood to spill into the surrounding tissue. Leakage of the blood into the surrounding tissue causes irreversible damage to that tissue. Hemorrhage can also be a result of physical injury, but that is less frequent in the arteries supplying the brain.

Thrombosis. Thrombosis occurs when a clot forms in a blood vessel in the brain. Clot formation during thrombosis is usually due to conditions that lead to atherosclerosis. When the clot reaches maximum size, blood supply is blocked, and the tissue that is normally supplied by that artery is damaged or killed.

Embolism. Embolism also results from a blood clot blocking a blood vessel. An embolism, as opposed to thrombosis, however, is the blocking of a vessel by a clot that was formed elsewhere in the body (such as in a vessel in the leg or arm) and that broke off and was carried through the bloodstream, eventually lodging in the lungs, heart, or brain.

Compression. An object in the brain—usually a tumor, a section of swollen tissue, or a blood clot from another vessel—can press on a blood vessel, exerting sufficient pressure to cut off the blood supply and restrict the flow of blood to outlying tissue.

Spasm. As a result of some diseases of the arteries, a blood vessel may briefly spasm, tightening and closing sufficiently to reduce or shut off blood flow. Some spasms are mild and of brief duration; permanent damage generally does not accompany a brief spasm. Others may be severe enough to cause a stroke.

SYMPTOMS

Symptoms of a stroke include difficulty in speaking, jumbled speech, or loss of the ability to speak; inability to understand the speech of others; sudden weakness or numbness in an arm or leg, in the face, or on one side of the body; loss of vision in one eye; dimming of eyesight in one or both eyes; brief episodes of double vision; dizziness or unsteadiness that cannot be attributed to another cause; a change in mental capacities, such as the sudden inability to remember the past or a sudden inability to calculate math; a change in personality; a pattern of headaches significantly different from the headaches you normally experience; difficulty in completing simple thought processes; or paralysis of some extremity (arm or leg), of the face, or one side of the body (such paralysis is generally permanent).[35]

ARE YOU AT RISK?

You run a risk of developing a stroke if you have high blood pressure; have had fleeting symptoms of minor strokes or have had a stroke before; have diabetes; are overweight; eat foods that are high in animal fats; have heart diseases of any kind; have atherosclerosis; or smoke.[36]

PREVENTION

The steps of prevention of stroke mirror the steps of prevention for other forms of heart disease:

- Get proper medical treatment. If you've had a series of minor strokes, or if you suspect that you might have suffered a slight stroke, see your doctor. He or she can help with treatment that may enable you to avoid having another stroke.
- Eat a well-balanced diet and restrict your intake of animal fats and foods that are high in cholesterol.
- Quit smoking.
- Reduce your weight to within a normal range for your height and frame.
- Reduce the amount of stress that you undergo.

ATHEROSCLEROSIS

By far the most common chronic disease affecting Americans, atherosclerosis is a slow, progressive disease that begins early in life and that generally goes undetected until middle or old age or until it causes a major medical problem.*

DEVELOPMENT OF ATHEROSCLEROSIS

Atherosclerosis deposits begin on the inside wall of a blood vessel—generally at a spot where the artery was damaged or injured previously in some way. Cholesterol, fats, and other fatty substances begin to stick to the spot on the artery wall, and the deposit begins to build. Other materials carried through the artery in the bloodstream adhere to the deposit, increasing its size and density.

Cells in the artery wall multiply, forming a collagen and a sticky substance that add to the size of the plaque and cause it to further attract blood platelets, substances from the body's blood-clotting system, and additional fats and cholesterols in the blood.

The interior of an artery is normally smooth and spacious, allowing for the free circulation of blood. Plaque due to the buildup of fats, cholesterol, collagen, and blood substances narrows the artery and cause its lining to become roughened, limiting its ability to conduct the flow of blood.

As the size of the plaque increases, the artery loses its flexibility, adding to the possibility that even more plaque will accumulate. Areas of the plaque that become irritated ulcerate, attract blood clots, and form scar tissue, thus further increasing in size.

If the plaque is allowed to continue growing, the artery eventually loses its elasticity completely, and the flow of blood is shut off due to blockage.

WHICH ARTERIES ARE AFFECTED?

Any artery in the body can be affected by plaque buildup. The ones that are most often affected, however, are the major arteries leading to the heart, lungs, brain, legs, and kidneys.

Plaque formation varies from person to person—and sometimes from artery to artery in the same person. In some instances the formation is rapid and is accompanied by a great deal of hardening of the artery; in other cases, plaque formation and buildup is slow and gradual, and little hardening takes place (younger people are less likely to experience as much hardening of the arteries as are older people).

*This section adapted from *Arteriosclerosis Fact Sheet,* 217/3285 (Washington, D.C.: U.S. Department of Health, Education and Welfare, Public Health Service, National Institutes of Health, 1978).

MAJOR CONSEQUENCES

Atherosclerosis doesn't affect just the arteries, unfortunately, its effects are felt throughout the body, and the severe damage or destruction of tissue it causes can lead to debilitation or death.

Some effects of atherosclerosis include the following:

Clots and pieces of the plaque may break off, being carried through the bloodstream until they lodge elsewhere in the same artery or in another artery. If the plaque is carried to a larger artery or to another place in the same artery, it will attach itself to the artery wall and begin anew the process of growth. If it is carried to a smaller artery, it can become lodged and completely block the blood flow (acting as an embolism).

Restriction of the blood supply to the heart results when the plaque formation is in the coronary arteries feeding the heart (a condition called ischemic heart disease). Portions of the heart muscle are deprived of oxygen and nutrients necessary for survival and proper functioning.

Angina pectoris, severe chest pain, results from inadequate blood flow to the heart, which is caused by plaque formation in coronary arteries. Different from the pain suffered during a heart attack, angina pectoris is a crushing, dull pain that generally lasts no longer than twenty minutes; over 2 million Americans currently suffer from angina pectoris.

Myocardial infarction (acute heart attack) can result if one or more of the coronary branches is abruptly shut off because of severe plaque buildup or because part of a large plaque deposit acts as an embolism and shuts off the blood supply. Sudden cardiac death, stroke, or congestive heart failure can result from interruption of the blood supply.

Intermittent claudication—transient episodes of pain and weakness, usually in the calf of the leg—results when plaque formation blocks arteries leading to the legs and results in inadequate blood supply. The pain is usually most severe during periods of physical exertion, and weakness may occur suddenly and without warning.

Gangrene, destruction of tissue, is a result of extreme degrees of blood deprivation. Once the tissue dies because of the blood deprivation, infection and putrefaction set in. Gangrene occurs only in the extremities (arms or legs) and is the result of plaque formation in the arteries leading to the extremities.

ARE YOU AT RISK?

You run a risk of developing atherosclerosis if

You have high levels of blood cholesterol. A difference of even thirty milligrams of cholesterol can increase your chance of developing atherosclerosis by over three times.

You have high blood pressure. High blood pressure (160/95 and higher) increases your risk of developing atherosclerosis by two to three times; the higher the blood pressure, the higher the risk of developing atherosclerosis.

You smoke. You increase your risk proportionately with the number of cigarettes you smoke each day. Once you have stopped smoking, it will take several years for your body to return to normal. Pipe and cigar smokers run a higher than normal risk, but not as high as the risk run by cigarette smokers.

You have diabetes. You run an extra risk if you are diabetic, female, and under fifty years of age.

You are obese. Obesity increases your risk because obese people tend to be less physically active, have higher levels of fats in the blood, have higher levels of sugars in the blood, and have high blood pressure.

You are older. Your risk grows greater as you grow older.

You are a man.

You have a family history of atherosclerosis—especially if your mother, father, sister, or brother developed atherosclerosis at an early age.

You take birth control pills.

You have a sedentary job and do not have a program of regular exercise, or you lead a generally sedentary life-style.

You undergo an excessive amount of stress.

PREVENTION
Take the steps necessary to protect yourself against other kinds of heart disease. Stop smoking. Eat properly, restricting your intake of cholesterol and animal fats. Exercise, and get the proper amount of rest to reduce the amount of stress you undergo. Take steps to control high blood pressure if you have it. Consult your doctor before using any method of oral contraception.

RHEUMATIC FEVER

Rheumatic fever usually strikes children between the ages of five and fifteen, and is always preceded by a streptococcal infection (strep throat). Not all strep infections lead to rheumatic fever, but those that go untreated or undetected are apt to progress to rheumatic fever.

Streptococcal bacteria from the original infection strike at the muscles of the heart, damaging them and inhibiting the heart's ability to perform to its fullest capacity. In extreme cases valves become scarred and deformed, allowing for leakage of blood between heart chambers.

EFFECTS OF RHEUMATIC FEVER
Although the death rate from rheumatic fever was once high due to the victim's inability to conquer infection, the discovery of penicillin and its widespread use has greatly reduced the number of children who die from a bout with rheumatic fever. The main concern now is with damage to the heart, which can result in later heart disease, serving to shorten life.

PREVENTION
The best prevention technique for rheumatic fever consists of prompt treatment of streptococcal infections.

Any sore throat that lasts longer than three days should be seen by a doctor and tested for possible streptococcus bacteria. If strep throat is confirmed, proper treatment—including vigorous therapy with penicillin or another antibiotic—should be undertaken.

Those who have had rheumatic fever once should be kept on a long-range program of penicillin therapy to prevent a recurrence of the disease.

CONGENITAL HEART DEFECTS

Congenital heart defects—those defects found in the heart at birth—result from abnormal development of the heart in the fetus. About eight out of every thousand children born in the United States have some kind of congenital heart defect.

CAUSES
Researchers have not yet isolated all of the factors that lead to congenital heart defects. One cause is disease or illness suffered by the mother during the first trimester of pregnancy; German measles are a particularly grim culprit. Other viral diseases are currently suspected, but medical confirmation is as yet unavailable. Heredity seems to be a factor in the likelihood of developing a congenital heart defect.[37]

KINDS OF DEFECTS
The most common defects of the heart manifest at birth include holes in the wall that divides the lower chambers of the heart, holes in the wall dividing the upper chambers of the heart, lack of closure between the artery delivering blood to the body and the artery delivering blood to the lungs, constriction or narrowing

of the largest artery in the body (the aorta), and transposition of the arteries delivering blood to the lungs and to the body (resulting in "blue babies," unable to get oxygenated blood).[38]

Death generally results if serious defects are not corrected; deaths in this case are usually due to the heart's inability to get an adequate blood supply or to the baby's inability to deliver oxygenated blood to organs and body tissues.[39]

Recent advances in microsurgery have enabled doctors to perform heart surgery on infants who are only hours old, thus enabling medical teams to reverse the damage done by an improperly formed heart.[40]

In some cases, the defects are not correctable but do not result in death. In these cases, the child generally has to exercise caution throughout life activities and to keep to a restricted diet.[41]

REDUCING THE RISK
OF HEART DISEASE

Heart disease is largely a preventable tragedy. We sentence our hearts—and ourselves—to death by the kinds of lives we lead. Very few factors that lead to heart disease—heredity, sex, and birth defects—are beyond our control.

You write your own ticket as far as a healthy heart is concerned. *You* have the ability to begin now to live the kind of life, to adopt the type of life-style, that will keep your heart beating strong, circulating life-giving nutrients throughout your body until you are silver-haired, bent with age, endowed with a proud heritage of a life fully lived. Or you have the ability to lead the kind of life-style that will make you an invalid, cut short your enjoyment of activities and adventure, or lead to your early death.

Take these measures to add years to your life:

Wage the battle of the bulge. Tighten your belt. Say no to second helpings. Get your weight down to where it is supposed to be, based on your height and your frame. Quit making your heart do overtime—every ounce of fat has to be supplied with blood vessels, and your heart has to pump blood to all of these vessels at least sixty or seventy times a minute. Give your heart a break—and maybe it will give you one, too.

Take it easy. We are a hurried generation: We rush from place to place, set impossible goals for ourselves, chew pencils and fingernails when we get behind schedule, get frantic when we get caught in traffic jams, find that there are never enough hours in the day. Relax. There *are* enough hours in the day; just learn to set realistic goals, to work on them one at a time, to finish one job before you move on to something else. Take advantage of your leisure time: Do things that you enjoy. And take breaks often. Quit worrying about what everybody else thinks of you. You're the only one who counts, and you should be happy with you. Not frustrated. And certainly not angry.

Create a stress-free environment. Surround yourself with things that you enjoy—people you enjoy being with, music you enjoy listening to, work you enjoy doing. Sure, we all have little stresses that we have to put up with, but they should be just that: little. Make some changes now; set about changing the major things in your life so that you can honestly say that you are happy most of the time.

Work at something you enjoy and that you can derive satisfaction from. Your job doesn't have to be the most glamorous one in the world. It doesn't even have to pay the best. It *does* have to provide a way for you to feel satisfied and rewarded. Work does *not* have to be a constant barrage of frustrations and miseries. If it is, consider a change. Now.

Get reacquainted with fruits and vegetables. And with whole grains, and with dairy products, and with meats and eggs and other sources of protein. In other words, eat a good, well-balanced variety of food. Kick the junk food habit. Reach for an apple instead of a donut. Your heart will thank you for it.

Watch what you drink. Alcohol hurts your heart. So does too much coffee, and too many carbonated beverages (they contain too much sugar). There are all kinds of good things to drink: milk, tomato juice, orange juice, water.

Get enough sleep. An adequate amount of sleep benefits your heart—and all of your other systems, too. In fact, sleep is one of the best health aids around. It gives your body a chance to rest, to recuperate, to heal. It's a respite from the day's stress and problems. It really is the pause that refreshes.

Quit smoking. Basically, smoking gums up the works. *All* the works. Every time you light up a cigarette, you shave a few minutes off your life. It's best if you never started smoking at all—but if you smoke now, *quit now.* Your body is an amazing machine; it will heal itself. Within a few years you will be just as healthy as if you never smoked—*if* you stop. Now.

Get enough exercise. Exercise doesn't have to be a boring routine of sit-ups, push-ups, and jumping jacks performed with dull regularity in the corner of your apartment kitchen. Exercise means running, jumping, bicycling, playing tennis, swimming, playing football, jogging, climbing, playing raquetball, dancing, jumping rope. You need some of it every day—a brisk walk to work would suffice—and you need some vigorous exercise at least once a week. Exercise has other good benefits besides strengthening your heart: It reduces your appetite so that you eat less, and you lose weight, and you are generally healthier all over.

In short, you can start right now—today—to do nice things for your heart. You can start to reverse the trend of heart disease in the United States. You can live and eat and sleep and move in such a way that you will be around to see the day when we are a healthier race of people, with stronger hearts and clearer minds.

Put your heart into it. It's all up to you.

SELF-EVALUATION TEST
PART I

Answer the following questions, and total your score from each.

1. Are you more than twenty-five pounds overweight? Add 3 points.

2. Are you more than thirty-five pounds overweight? Add 6 points.

3. Is your diastolic blood pressure 90 to 100? Add 3 points.

4. Is your diastolic blood pressure over 100? Add 6 points.

5. Do you smoke? Add 3 points.

6. Do you smoke more than two packs of cigarettes a day? Add 6 points.

7. Is your life-style sedentary? Add 3 points.

8. Does someone in your family have diabetes? Add 3 points.

9. Do you have diabetes? Add 6 points.

10. Did either of your parents or a brother or sister have a heart attack before the age of sixty? Add 3 points.

11. Do you have a high level of cholesterol (over 250)? Add 6 points.

12. Do you have a slightly elevated level of cholesterol (210 to 250)? Add 3 points.

13. Did your last electrocardiogram show any abnormalities? Add 3 points.

SCORING

If you did not have to answer yes to any of the foregoing questions, your life-style and family history are such that you run a low risk of developing heart disease. If your score was 9 to 15 points, you run a moderate risk of developing heart disease of some kind. If your score was 18 to 36 points, you run an extremely high risk of developing heart disease.

PART II

Answer the following questions and total the appropriate score to find your risk factor of suffering a heart attack.*

1. Age

11–20	1 point
21–30	2 points
31–40	3 points
41–50	4 points
51–60	5 points
61 and older	6 points

2. Number of close relatives who died of coronary heart disease before the age of 55

1	3 points
2 or more	5 points

3. Weight

Normal	0 points
10–15 pounds overweight	1 point
15–25 pounds overweight	2 points
25–35 pounds overweight	4 points
More than 35 pounds overweight	6 points

4. Saturated fat in diet

None	0 points
Less than 15 percent	2 points
30 percent (average American diet)	4 points
Over 40 percent	6 points

5. Cholesterol level (check with your doctor)

150–90	0 points
191–220	1 point
221–50	2 points
251–80	3 points
281–300	4 points
301–340	5 points
More than 340	6 points

*Adapted from "Heart Attack Risk Profile," *Life and Health*, October 1976, pp. 22–23.

6. Blood pressure

100/60	0 points
120/70	1 point
140/80	2 points
160/90	3 points
175/100	4 points
190/110	5 points
200/120	6 points

7. Cigarette smoking

None	0 points
10 or less per day	2 points
11–20 per day	3 points
21–30 per day	4 points
31–40 per day	5 points
More than 40 per day	6 points

8. Personality type

Type B (cheerful, easygoing)	0 points
Type A (driving, competitive)	6 points

9. Exercise

Frequent hard physical work	0 points
Sedentary work, regular exercise	3 points
Sedentary work, no exercise	6 points

SCORING

If your score is:	Your overall risk is:
Up to 8	Very low
8-19	Low
19-30	Average
30-43	High
Over 43	Extremely high

REFERENCES

[1]American Heart Association, *Heart Facts 1978* (Dallas: American Heart Association, Inc., 1977), pamphlet no. 55-005-B, p. 2.

[2]This and the following from Paul Kezdi, *You and Your Heart* (New York: Atheneum Publishers, 1978), pp. 3–18.

[3]American Heart Association, *Heart Facts 1978*, p. 2.

[4]Ibid.

[5]Theodore Irwin, *Watch Your Blood Pressure,* rev. ed. (Bethesda, Md.: U.S. Department of Health, Education and Welfare, National Institutes of Health, Public Affairs Commission, 1976), pamphlet no. 483A, p. 3.

[6]Ibid.

[7]Ibid., p. 4.

[8]*What Every Woman Should Know About High Blood Pressure* (Bethesda, Md.: U.S. Department of Health, Education and Welfare, National Institutes of Health, 1974), DHEW publication no. (NIH) 75-733, p. 1; Irwin, *Watch Your Blood Pressure,* p. 12.

[9]Irwin, *Watch Your Blood Pressure,* p. 9.

[10]Ibid., p. 13.

[11]Ibid., p. 14.

[12]Ibid.

[13]Ibid.

[14]Milton G. Crane, "High Blood Pressure," *Life and Health*, July 1976, p. 14.

[15]Ibid.

[16]Ibid.

[17]Ibid., p. 15.

[18]Ibid.

[19]Ibid.

[20]"A Look at High Blood Pressure," *The Harvard Medical School Health Letter,* 4, no. 9 (July 1979), p. 1.

[21]"Salt and High Blood Pressure," *Consumer Reports,* March 1979, pp. 147–49.

[22]J. A. Scharffenberg, "What You Need to Know About High Blood Pressure," *Life and Health,* December 1978, p. 5.

[23]Ibid.

[24]*What Every Woman Should Know About High Blood Pressure,* p. 1.

[25]Ross and O'Rourke, *Understanding the Heart,* p. 88.

[26]"What Is a Heart Attack?" *Life and Health,* October 1976, p. 12.

[27]American Heart Association, *Heart Facts 1978,* p. 4.

[28] "Early Warnings of a Heart Attack," card T.15135, Metropolitan Life Insurance Company.

[29] Ibid.

[30] *Congestive Heart Failure Fact Sheet* (Washington, D.C.: U.S. Department of Health, Education and Welfare, Public Health Service, National Institutes of Health, 1976), pub. no. 20.3202.H3518, p. 1.

[31] James V. Warren, "Understanding Chronic Heart Failure," *Drug Therapy,* June 1978, p. 81.

[32] *Congestive Heart Failure Fact Sheet,* pp. 2–3.

[33] "Stroke," *American Druggist,* November 1977, p. 41.

[34] *Cerebral Vascular Disease and Strokes* (Washington, D.C.: U.S. Department of Health, Education and Welfare, Public Health Service, National Institutes of Health, 1972), pub. no. 0-489-484, pp. 5–6.

[35] Ibid., p. 7; "Stroke," p. 43.

[36] *Cerebral Vascular Disease and Strokes,* p. 9.

[37] *Inborn (Congenital) Heart Defects* (Bethesda, Md.: U.S. Department of Health, Education and Welfare, Public Health Service, National Institutes of Health, 1976), DHEW publication no. (NIH) 76-1085, pp. 2–3.

[38] Ibid., pp. 1–2.

[39] Ibid.

[40] Ibid.

[41] Ibid.

CANCER
THE NUMBER-TWO KILLER

According to recent statistics, cancer will strike approximately two out of three American families. The victim might be your father. Your child. Your grandmother. Your sister. Your wife. Maybe even you.

Of every three people who get cancer one will be saved. Two will die.

The tragedy lies in the fact that about 117,000 of those who died of cancer as recently as 1980 could have been saved by earlier treatment—and that earlier treatment can only result from earlier detection. Of those three who will die from cancer, one can be saved by early detection. The other two can be saved when medical research discovers the keys that will unlock the mysteries of cancer.

What does all of this mean to you?

You've seen the television and magazine advertisements beckoning you to learn cancer's seven warning signals. They mean business: You need to learn to recognize certain symptoms in your own body. You need to know when it's time to see a doctor.

There are other important things, too. You can learn whether you are a high-risk individual: Exactly how likely are you to contract cancer? Do you have weaknesses that may predispose you to developing cancer? Might you be susceptible to cancer of the breast? Colon? Lung? Thyroid?

You can learn the characteristics of cancer—what causes it, how it spreads. You can learn what things you can do today, and for the rest of your life, to lessen your chances of being one of those who suffer and die from what has become the nation's number-two killer (second only to heart disease).

At the present time, at least one hundred different kinds of cancer have been classified by their appearance under the microscope and by the site of the body in which they develop. Some grow slowly, destroying neighboring tissue

67

by limited spread; others spread rapidly to different parts of the body, involving a number of organs and often causing death in a different body site from where they originated.[1]

Cancer strikes people of all nationalities, all ages, and all social and economic classes. It strikes married people and single people. No one is completely immune, but everyone can learn the early warning signs and can be diagnosed early. Many can survive. In fact, with all the current knowledge and experience available to medical technicians, about one-half of all cancer victims should be saved. It is up to us to make that possibility a reality.

THE NATURE OF CANCER

Cancer, a word derived from the Greek word for crab *(karkinos)*, stands for a large group of diseases that afflict man and animals. Cancer can arise in any organ in the body; its main characteristic is an abnormal, seemingly unrestricted growth of body cells. The resultant mass—or tumor—compresses, invades, and destroys adjacent normal tissues. Sometimes cancer cells break off and leave the original mass and are carried by the blood or lymph to distant sites of the body, where they set up secondary growths *(metastases)*, further attacking and destroying the organs involved.

In cancer something in the normal body processes goes wrong. From birth to death, the normal living organism is constantly changing. It grows, degenerates, sustains injury and repairs the damage, reproduces, transforms digested food into energy, and adapts itself to its environment. All of this activity involves the death and orderly replacement of millions of cells every day.

Normal cells multiply, differentiate into specialized individual types, and become organized, integrated units of tissues and systems.

Cancer cells, though, continue to multiply beyond the limits designed for normal cells. They lack organization and proper differentiation. What is really a normal body process—the process of control that governs the repair of skin incisions, the healing of broken bones, and the replacement of lost blood—becomes deranged. Normally, those healing and regeneration processes cease once the damage has been corrected. In some cases, though, for an unknown reason, that regeneration becomes prolific. The regeneration does not stop when the damage is repaired; instead, the body is overrun by wildly growing cells: cancer.

Some evidence indicates that the body may treat cancer as it does any invading organism: It may actually attempt to develop an antibody-antigen to fight the invading cancer cells. If so, this discovery could lead to further discoveries that would aid medical researchers in developing helps to the body's response to cancer.

Those invading cancer cells eventually become a new growth, originally called a *neoplasm* and now commonly referred to as a *tumor*. Understanding the workings of a tumor is vital to understanding the disease process of cancer.

Tumors fall into two major groups: benign (those that grow slowly, never spread, contain cells that resemble the normal cells in the adjacent organ, and are contained in a fibrous capsule), and malignant (those that invade other tissues, grow rapidly, contain a number of abnormal cells of various sizes and shapes, and are rarely contained in a fibrous capsule). If benign tumors are promptly identified and treated, they are usually cured. But there are hazards connected to malignant tumors: They invade the surrounding tissues and they spread to involve other tissues.[2]

Metastasis, the spread of tumors (usually malignant) to distant sites in the body unique from the area of origin, involves five steps:

1. When the cells from the primary tumor invade the tissue immediately surrounding the tumor, the invading cells penetrate blood and lymph vessels.
2. Tumor cell clumps (emboli), composed of either single or multiple cells, are released into the lymph or blood circulatory system.
3. As the emboli circulate, they are trapped in the small, narrow blood vessels that pass through the body's organs.
4. The emboli penetrate the walls of the vessels and penetrate into adjacent tissue of the organ. There they multiply.
5. The cells multiply until they have formed a new tumor (called a secondary tumor). The process now begins all over again.

A critical factor in metastasis is the malignant tumors' rate of growth and their invasive properties (their ability to invade into adjacent tissues, which depends on a host of complex factors involving both the tumor and the organ tissue that is being invaded). Malignant cells themselves have some unique characteristics. They usually lack structural features and distinctive functions. Many malignant cells divide rapidly; the continuous multiplication of the cells in a confined area of the body results in pressure within the tissue. First the blood supply is interrupted; subsequently the tissue is destroyed.

But the rate of cell division and multiplication is not always needed for the invasion process; some tumor cells that grow very slowly (such as malignant breast tumors) invade rapidly and easily despite their slow growth. Even normal cells can sometimes be invasive; for instance, white blood cells invade tissues, but do not divide inside those tissues. Even some rapidly dividing cells—such as those required for healing of wounds and for regeneration of tissue material—are not invasive.

So invasion does not depend on the cell's multiplication. On what, then, *does* it depend? First of all, malignant cells are not sticky like other cells are. They are easily separated from one another, and can easily invade other tissues. This lack of stickiness is probably due to a lack of calcium on the cell surface. (Even this quality is not unique to cancer cells, however; certain normal cells—such as white blood cells or cells in the developing fetus—are completely mobile.)

Some studies indicate that malignant cells may secrete an attractant composed of a protein that induces other circulating tumor cells to enter the tissues around the tumor.

The tumor causes damage and destruction of the surrounding organ cells in two ways. First, the pressure cuts off blood supply and results in deterioration of the tissues. Second, a toxic substance is produced by, stored in, and secreted by invasive tumor cells; that toxic substance causes destruction of surrounding tissues.

A second major factor in metastasis is the way the cancerous cells spread throughout the body. That spreading process depends on how long the person has had the disease, as well as which way the cells are spread throughout the body: by direct extension (or transplantation), transmission through the lymphatic system, or transmission through the bloodstream.

Tumors that grow into or that invade surrounding body tissues often release cells that travel freely to distant organ surfaces, where they develop into new tumors. This shedding process is called *direct extension;* a good example is a tumor of the ovary that sheds cells into the abdominal cavity, where they can become implanted on the uterus, the intestinal tract, or other abdominal organs. Most tumors of the central nervous system are spread in this way; few enter the lymph or blood systems, although some are spread through cerebrospinal fluid.

The *lymphatic system* is the most common pathway for spread of malignant tumors. Lymph, a fluid that collects in lymphatic capillaries, flows into larger vessels, and passes through the lymph nodes, eventually enters the bloodstream through ducts located in the neck.

There are several ways, then, that a lymphatic transmission can occur. Tumor cells might invade a draining lymph node, where they can enter the lymph system and be transported to a distant site. Or a tumor may invade a lymph vessel, where emboli may break off and circulate through the lymph system, eventually becoming lodged in a distant narrow vessel.

Studies have shown that tumor cells readily move between the lymph and the blood systems, so it is difficult to tell exactly what role each plays in the metastasis process.

Even when they are not invaded by cancer themselves, the lymph nodes react to a cancerous tumor that is in their vicinity. Lymph nodes located near a primary tumor, for instance, often become enlarged—due to what scientists suspect is an immunity reaction.

Thin-walled veins offer the most common pathway for cancer cells through

70

the *bloodstream;* the arteries, with their elastic and collagen walls, provide prime resistance to invasion by cancer emboli.

Cancer cells that do invade the blood vessels can either become lodged at the invasion site and proliferate there (causing clots made of blood protein to form around the actively growing tumor) or be carried away in the bloodstream to lodge at a distant site.

Generation of tumor emboli is probably a continuous process, and the bloodstream is probably used throughout the life of the tumor. Most malignant tumors have a well-established blood supply, including their own multiple, thin-walled vessels. Because of this, a sudden jolt to the tumor—such as the sudden change of pressure that occurs in the veins when you cough—could release sudden showers of tumor emboli that would then enter the bloodstream and be carried to another site. Even procedures that doctors use to diagnose and locate the tumors can cause this sudden release of cancer emboli to enter the bloodstream.

All cancer emboli that enter the bloodstream do not lodge and become tumors. Most emboli do not survive to develop into new growths because of the hazards they face in the bloodstream: (1) blood turbulence, (2) the body's defense mechanisms, and (3) thick-walled arteries that do not enable the emboli to implant and work through into surrounding organ tissue. The cancer cells' success in developing into new tumors depends on how long the primary tumor has been growing—which in turn determines what size the cancer emboli are. Some specialists estimate that only about 0.01 percent of all circulating emboli develop into new growths; some victims have survived for years after their primary tumors were removed, even though they still had emboli circulating through their bloodstream.

Metastases are found more frequently in some organs than in others primarily because those organs are more richly supplied by veins or they provide a pooling place for venous blood. The lung and liver are the two most common sites to be affected by metastasis; the bones are also commonly involved. In contrast, cancer seldom (if ever) metastasizes to the spleen, skeletal muscle, cartilage, or thyroid. Tumors in those locations are almost always primary tumors.

What determines whether an embolism that lodges in an organ will develop into a new growth? Much depends on the condition of the organ and on how favorable its "soil" is to the growth of the cancer cell. There are some factors—including blood clot formation, direct injury to the organ, altered blood flow, or existing disease in the organ—that can make it easier for the cancer cell to survive and grow. For instance, a liver that has sustained blunt injury or that has been diseased by cirrhosis is more likely to offer an inviting-host atmosphere to a cancer cell than is a liver that is healthy and strong.

Once a cancer cell implants and begins to grow, new blood vessels are formed that begin at once to nourish the tumor. For some reason, a tumor actually stimulates the surrounding tissue to generate a network of new blood vessels that supply it with food.

There are a number of factors that can increase metastasis—among them are hormones, radiation, and physical injury. In some instances physical injury can make a host tissue or organ more susceptible to the growth and survival of cancer cells that may metastasize to the area or that may already exist there. Physical injury itself, though, does not cause the creation of cancer cells where none already exist.

CAUSES OF CANCER

No one knows exactly what causes cancer, or whether the same factor is responsible for causing different kinds of cancer. If we knew exactly what caused cancer, of course, we would be much closer to finding an effective cure.

Some researchers suspect a virus.[3] Some kinds of cancer appear to be hereditary—or to be influenced by hereditary factors—such as cancer of the eye, breast, and intestine.[4] Other kinds of cancer appear to be caused by environmental factors.

Whatever their cause, it is apparent that cancer cells grow slowly over a period of years—and that they could be detected and treated long before symptoms appear. Their causes appear to be as varied as the kinds of cancers, but there are some factors that seem to be definite:

Condition of long-term irritation. This includes extensive and frequent exposure to sunlight, which is believed to be a primary cause of skin cancer; continued irritation of the lip by the hot steam of a pipe, which causes cancer of the lip in pipe smokers; constant irritation of the cheek from chewing betel nuts (a common practice in Southeast Asia); irritation to a pigmented mole caused by friction from a belt, brassiere strap, or suspenders; or cancer of the tongue caused by frequent and long-lasting ulcerations.

Exposure to specific agents. Cigarette smoking, painting with luminous paint, exposure to X rays, and occupational hazards of asbestos work have all been linked to cancer that develops in various body organs. Whatever they may be, agents that are suspected to cause cancer are called *carcinogens*. Generally they are chemical, environmental, or radioactive in nature. Most are environmental: Today's industry and technology have turned us into caged canaries who, through illness, herald the presence of highly toxic chemicals introduced into our environment.[5]

Benign tumors that become malignant. A prime example of this phenomenon is that of leukoplakia, white patches on the mouth (benign) that eventually become malignant cancer of the mouth. Those tumors or conditions that may lead to cancer are termed *precancerous,* or *premalignant.* Inroads are being accomplished in treating such precancerous conditions (and in identifying them earlier) before they become cancerous.

Hormones. Evidence currently strongly suggests that hormones are in some way involved in the development of certain cancers. Cancer of the breast is a good example.

There is still a great deal to be learned about what causes cancer. Much seems to be dependent on the individual body; for instance, some people who have precancerous conditions never develop cancer. In others cancer may develop suddenly, without any identifiable predisposing factors.

Researchers recently postulated that there may be a "cancer-prone personality."[6] The Third International Symposium on the Detection and Prevention of Cancer reported from New York City that this may be especially true of women—that women who go through life either grimly suppressing their emotions or venting their feelings in hostile ways are much more prone to developing cancer than are women who use moderation in expressing their sentiments.

There are two—opposite—personality traits that seem to be common to cancer victims: extreme suppression or extreme violent outburst. Both those who "bottle up" their feelings and those who have frequent temper outbursts seem to run a higher risk of developing cancer—especially cancer of the breast. Studies conducted by British and American doctors revealed that those who developed cancer have possessed the same character traits throughout their entire adult lives—and some had even possessed them as children.

In other tests conducted at Memorial Sloan-Kettering Cancer Center in New York City cancer victims were found to have unusual self-control: They were serious, sober, diligent, and practical. Most were overcontrolled, especially when it came to expressing their emotions. According to some medical specialists extensive research in this area could pave the way for psychological screening of the general population, perhaps making us able someday to predict those who might develop cancer years in advance by asking a series of simple personality questions.

There may be another personality-linked determinant to cancer: A report from Johns Hopkins University's Oncology center revealed that women who were docile in accepting their breast cancer were more likely to die; those who fought the doctors, the treatments, and who viewed the disease and all of its ramifications in a negative way lived longer. Why? They had more vigor. They had the energy to fight back.

ENVIRONMENTAL CANCERS

Many carcinogens, then, originate in our environment; some estimate that the figure may be as high as 90 percent of all cancers. Federal agencies such as the Environmental Protection Agency (EPA) and the Federal Drug Administration (FDA) are currently embroiled in controversies trying to establish a definition for "acceptable levels" of all kinds of environmental pollutants, from industrial waste to pesticides. The National Institute for Occupational Safety and Health (NIOSH) is also concerned about environmental pollutants that affect people on the job, and they report that there are 390,000 new cases each year of job-related cancers.[7]

We can fit a number of carcinogens into the environmental category: chemicals, general pollutants, radiation, food and drink, and drugs. Some of these carcinogens may not cause cancer, but may increase the risk.

CHEMICALS
In an effort to control the number of poisonous chemicals in the environment, the government in 1976 passed the Toxic Substances Control Act, legislation that required more rigorous testing and controls for use of new chemicals. The legislation may have little effect on the carcinogens among the chemicals currently used by people, though. Why? Because a number of those carcinogens are in chemicals manufactured and distributed prior to the 1976 passage of the law.

One important chemical carcinogen developed prior to 1976 is PCBs—polychlorinated biphenyls. They've been on the market for almost forty years and are used in electrical transformers, capacitors, paints, inks, paper, plastics, adhesives, sealants, and hydraulic fluid.

Because they were concerned about the carcinogenic qualities of the PCBs, their principal manufacturer, the Monsanto Company, voluntarily restricted their production, but they still abound in our environment because of the number of products produced during the last forty years. For instance, the World Trade Center in New York City has 250,000 fluorescent light fixtures, each filled with PCB to reduce the fire hazard.[8] Unfortunately, too, PCBs do not readily break down into nature; the only way to destroy them is with unusually high temperatures and rapid incineration. One researcher believes that there are 300,000 tons of PCBs in junkyards in this country alone; 60,000 tons may have already been dumped into American waters.

As a result, traces of PCBs have been found in mother's milk, in almost all human tissue samples collected in this country, in the flesh of fish from freshwater lakes and streams, in penguin eggs collected in Antarctica, and in animals captured in such remote spots as Greenland. It is a widespread problem indeed.

What are the effects of PCB? Cancer is one. There are others: mental retardation, reproductive disorders, skin lesions, liver problems, hair loss, and metabolic disorders. And consider this: The average breast-fed baby is getting ten times more PCBs through its mother's milk than the amount the FDA considers safe.

Another similar chemical—PBBs (polybrominated biphenyls)—have effects much like those of PCBs. But the PBBs are five times more toxic. And we recently discovered that the chemical was accidentally mixed in feed for cattle, hogs, and chickens. Countless numbers of people were exposed through at least 500 Michigan farms.

GENERAL POLLUTANTS

Air pollution, which obliterates the skylines in many American cities, may also be linked to lung cancer.[9] These air pollutants come from industrial waste and from automobile exhaust—both of which contain carcinogenic elements.

Even contamination of the water supplies can cause cancer. But there may be an even worse danger: Recent studies reveal that the chemical used to *purify* water, chlorine, may interact with other substances to produce carcinogens.[10] It's hard to decide which is worse—the infectious bacteria or the purifiers. One glass of tap water taken from a New Orleans household contained sixty-six organic chemicals; of those eight were highly toxic potential carcinogens.

Then there are the pesticides, herbicides, and fungicides—a number of them leading carcinogens.

RADIATION

As will be discussed later in this chapter, X rays, radium paint, and radioactive fallout all act as potentially lethal carcinogens. And the most convincing evidence that ionizing radiation causes cancer was obtained in studies of the survivors of Hiroshima and Nagasaki—persons who developed a critically high rate of leukemia.

FOOD AND DRINK

Let's start with the basics: drinking water. Besides chlorine, there are other carcinogens in water; fluoridation was recently pinpointed as a probable serious carcinogen.[11]

Complex chemical interactions in the foods we eat cause a number of those foods (and food additives) to be carcinogenic.[12] Two of the most dangerous food additives are sodium nitrate and sodium nitrite—used in bacon, ham, and smoked foods and naturally present in some water supplies. Nitrates in smoked fish have been linked to a high incidence of stomach cancer in Japan.

The nitrites are also related to another risk: The substances become volatile during cooking. It was recently claimed that griddle-fried hamburgers may contain a carcinogen.[13] The studies accompanying the hamburger statistics indicated that the same carcinogens may be present in other cooked meats, too—not just beef.

75

The worst risk from foods and drink is an indirect—but important—one: Diets high in fat have been definitely linked to cancer. Those people who eat foods high in fat and low in fiber run a definite risk of developing several kinds of cancer.[14] Low-fiber diets cause cancer of the bowel, colon, and stomach; diets high in fat have been shown to cause cancer of the breast, ovary, uterus, and prostate.

Among the leading carcinogens used in food is Dimethylaminoazobenzene, used to color margarine yellow, which has been linked to cancer of the liver.

Alcohol consumption also bears impact. Heavy drinkers run the risk of developing cancer of the mouth, throat, esophagus, larynx, and liver. The risk is even worse for those heavy drinkers who also smoke.

DRUGS

Because drugs are taken in relatively large doses, researchers are more concerned with them than with the environmental or chemical additives we are exposed to. Two striking examples are the high rates of cancer directly related to DES (diethylstilbesterol) and other estrogens when used in treating pregnancy-related problems.

Even the birth control pill—currently taken by millions of American women—has been tentatively linked to certain kinds of cancer, especially cancer of the breast. However, the data are still sketchy and controversial.

Drugs used to prevent rejection of human transplanted organs have also been shown to cause cancer, especially lymphatic cancer. Other drugs used in the treatment of psoriasis, acne, and sore throats may cause cancer. Even aspirin, if used improperly, may be carcinogenic. And the list goes on: DES, used by many women in the 1960s to prevent miscarriage and which has caused vaginal cancer in their offspring; vinyl chloride, which causes cancer of the liver; saccharin; and DDT.

INCIDENCE OF CANCER

About 370,000 Americans die of cancer every year; its incidence rises about 2 percent every year. Currently more than 1,000 people die each day from cancer in this country alone—that's one every ninety seconds. Over 1 million Americans are currently undergoing treatment for some form of cancer.

More men than women die of cancer. The most fatal cancers in women are breast, colon and rectum, uterus, lung, pancreas, stomach, and leukemia; those account for over 70 percent of all cancer deaths in women. Leading cancer killers in men include lung, colon and rectum, prostate, stomach, pancreas, leukemia, and bladder. In both men and women combined, lung cancer is the leading killer.

More than half of all cancer deaths occur in victims over sixty-five years of age, but about 3,500 children under the age of fifteen die of cancer each year. If the current mortality and cancer incidence rates remain at their present level, the chance that a person now under the age of twenty will develop cancer at some time during his or her life is about one in four for males and slightly higher for females.

What about those who are able to arrest their cancers? How many will suffer a recurrence? The exact figures are unknown, but according to medical research scientists at the University of Liege in Belgium, that recurrence may be predictable and, therefore, treatable.[15]

SPECIFIC KINDS
OF CANCER

There are twelve most prevalent sites for new cancers to develop, according to the National Conference's Third National Cancer Survey. You should be aware of each of these, including their warming signals and safeguards you can take to prevent your developing such cancers.

BREAST

The leading cause of cancer death in women, breast cancer, claims over 30,000 victims each year in the United States. About 90,000 new cases are reported in this country each year; figures are similar for other highly developed countries.[16]

Many lumps that develop in the breast are not cancerous; about 65 to 80 percent of them are benign. While the death rate from breast cancer is high in this country, it is markedly low in the USSR, Japan, parts of eastern Asia, Africa, and the Carribean. Mortality from breast cancer is highest among Jewish women and among women of upper social and economic groups.[17]

Perhaps even more than in other kinds of cancers, early detection is the key to survival and cure of breast cancer. You can increase your chances of avoiding serious complications if you understand the nature of the breast and if you understand what breast cancer is and what you can do about it.[18]

Human milk is the food that contains all the proper elements essential for a human infant's growth and development; the breast is a highly specialized gland that produces human milk. That gland is enclosed in a specially shaped vessel that was designed and located for optimum convenience of both the mother and the child.

The interior of the breast is laced with a network of ducts that end in small lobules, where the milk is produced from substances derived from the blood. Those ducts in turn lead to the nipple, where it can be used by the infant.

Your breast isn't confined to just the front of your chest; it reaches into the armpit and over to the breast bone. That's an important fact to know as you try to understand the nature and treatment of breast cancer. In the armpit and under the breastbone are numerous lymph glands—which, as you may know, act as filters and traps for harmful substances in the body, including cancerous cells.

Breasts change, of course, as they grow and develop, but they continue to change throughout life in response to hormonal changes, menstruation, pregnancy, and the menopause.

Breast cancer is not as common as the symptoms of breast cancer— tenderness, swelling, pain, and nipple discharge—which are frequent and attributable to a number of causes. But the fact that they are frequent and that they many times do *not* signal cancer does not mean that you should ignore them if they do occur. You should arrange *immediately* for an examination by a physician if you notice any of these signs or if you detect a lump of any kind. They will probably not mean that you have cancer, but if you do have cancer, your early and prompt medical attention will probably save your life.

You should be aware of the fact that many conditions in the breast can cause lumps and masses of hard tissue to develop; most of these lumps and masses are benign, but they nevertheless need to be surgically removed to preserve the healthy condition of the breast. If you have a lump, and your doctor recommends surgery, it does not necessarily mean that you have cancer.

The breast is in an exposed position on the body, and it sustains frequent injury, stimulation, and manipulation. Do any of those cause cancer? No. The delicate breast gland is actually protected by a layer of fat that surrounds and pads it, a tough fibrous tissue that surrounds it, and the layer of skin that completely covers it. Sometimes you might be struck or otherwise injured, and the tiny capillaries beneath your skin may rupture and begin to bleed, causing dark purple discolorations. This is alarming, but it does not cause cancer. Neither does the frequent manipulation of the breasts that may occur as a result of lovemaking or breast feeding. You may also occasionally suffer from an inflammation, irritation, or infection that involves your breast; these do not cause cancer, either.

So what *does* cause breast cancer? Scientists are not sure, but they *can* clearly recognize a breast cancer cell under the microscope, and a great deal is known about the behavior of breast cancer cells.

As discussed earlier, cancer cells are not governed by the same rules that govern other cells in the body: They are loosely structured and they wander about at will, establishing new cancer sites at other places in the body.

In breast cancer the body is able to keep the cancer localized for a certain period of time. Cells that break from the main tumor are destroyed by the body's immune systems; the cancer is contained in the breast during that time.

After some time, however—a time period that varies with each individual—the body defenses give up, and the cancer cells that break away from the primary tumor are able to survive and establish new colonies in other organs. At that point, the cancer is difficult to control and leads to widespread tissue destruction.

It is critical, then, that the cancer is diagnosed while it is still contained within the breast; it is critical that the cancer be removed (through surgery) before it spreads to any other part of the body. That is why early detection is so important.

Six factors affect the frequency of breast cancer:

Age. The risk of developing breast cancer increases with age. A woman who is seventy years old is ten times more likely to develop breast cancer than is a woman who is forty years old. Incidentally, although it is not common, men can also develop breast cancer.

Geographic location. Women and men are most likely to develop breast cancer if they live in the United States, northern Europe, Canada, and Israel. Those in Japan, China, South America, or Africa develop it about one-sixth as often.

Ethnicity. Blacks and Puerto Ricans are less likely to develop breast cancer than are whites or Jews. Whites and Jewish people in high economic subgroups are at a particularly high risk.

Family background. If your mother, sister, or aunt had breast cancer, you run a significantly higher risk of developing it, especially if more than one member of your family had breast cancer.

Number of children borne. If you have several children, or if you have a hysterectomy involving removal of your ovaries before you turn thirty-five, you have less chance of developing breast cancer than a woman who has never had children.

Age at motherhood. If you carry a child full term before you are twenty, you develop a strong protection against breast cancer that will continue throughout your life—even if you never have another baby. No one knows why, but this factor helps explain why women in some underdeveloped countries—who bear children at a much earlier age—have a lower incidence of breast cancer.

It was once believed that nursing a child protects a woman against breast cancer. Recent findings, however, demonstrate that nursing has no bearing on whether a woman will develop breast cancer.

There are some additional factors that may influence the development of breast cancer; some medical technicians claim that use of oral contraceptives and use of hormones after menopause may contribute significantly to the incidence of breast cancer. Such claims are still a subject of controversy. If you are taking any form of hormone treatment, however, it is a good idea to have a regular breast examination by your physician to help detect any problems.

As mentioned, you may at some time in your life develop symptoms that resemble breast cancer. One of the most common of these is the lump, or cyst. Most occur prior to menopause; many contain fluid, which can easily be drained by a needle inserted into the cyst (a method that does not require surgery). Others need to be surgically removed. Whatever the makeup of the cysts, they do not cause cancer and probably do not lead to its development in the breast, either.

Another cancerlike symptom is nipple discharge. Some women, because of the irritation to the ducts, develop a watery discharge from the nipple accompanied by neither pain nor any other discomfort. A number of conditions may cause this discharge, and they may be completely unrelated to cancer.

You must be completely aware of these symptoms, though, even though most will not turn out to be cancer, you *must* be examined by your doctor anyway. This is the time when you can take an aggressive step toward your own protection against breast cancer.

There are two kinds of examination: one that you perform yourself (hopefully once a month), and one that is performed by your doctor or other medical technician.

SELF-EXAMINATION

The next time you go to your doctor, have him or her demonstrate breast self-examination so you can make sure you are doing it correctly. Also ask to have the breast's structure explained. The first time you perform a breast self-examination, you will feel lumps, masses, and ridges of tissue: No one's breast is simply a jellylike mass. Have your doctor show you which of these are normal. Be aware of the fact that your breast will vary in texture from year to year and sometimes during a single month. If you are regular and thorough in your breast self-examination, you will be able to feel these changes and will be able to tell if something abnormal begins to happen. If you *do* feel a lump that should not be there, don't panic. And, for your own sake, don't let fear keep you away from your doctor's office. Make an appointment and keep it. Your doctor will be able to tell you what the lump is—and may be able to save your life.

Breast self-examination can lead to earlier detection of breast cancer and, therefore, to a higher rate of cure. You should examine your breasts regularly, once a month, at the same time each month; the best time to do it is immediately following your period, because your breasts will be less tender and swollen than they will be before or during your period. If you have had a hysterectomy, have completed menopause, or for some other reason do not have a menstrual period, examine your breasts on the first day of each month.

Follow this procedure:[19]

IN THE SHOWER
While you take a bath or shower, you will be able to glide your fingers over your wet skin easily. With your fingers flat against your skin, move them gently over every part of each breast. Use your right hand to examine your left breast, and your left hand to examine your right breast. Check for any kind of a thickening, lump, or hard knot that your doctor has not confirmed as a normal part of breast structure.

IN FRONT OF A MIRROR
Look at your breasts in the mirror while you hold your arms down to your sides. Then raise your arms (both of them) high over your head and look at your breasts again. You need to look carefully and see if there is any swelling in either breast, if there are any contour changes in either breast, if any of the skin is dimpling, or if there are any changes in the nipples.

Rest your palms on your hips and press down firmly so that your chest muscles flex. Don't worry if your breasts don't match exactly; few women's do. By regularly performing this examination, though, you will learn what is normal for you, and you will be able to tell when a change in contour does occur.

LYING DOWN
Lie down on your back; begin by examining your right breast. Put a pillow or a folded towel or blanket under your right shoulder; put your right hand under your head. This posture distributes your breast tissue more evenly across your chest wall. Use your left hand for the examination; with your fingers flat against your skin, press gently in small circular motions around an imaginary clock face. Start at the outermost top of your right breast (twelve o'clock); move to one o'clock, then two o'clock, and so on around your breast back to where you started (twelve o'clock). You will feel a ridge of firm tissue in the lower curve of each breast; it is normal.

Now move in an inch from the original circle you just examined. Complete the same kind of examination, moving in one inch toward the nipple each time. A thorough examination will require at least three more circles. Be sure you examine the portion that lies underneath the nipple.

Now repeat the same procedure on your left breast, with the pillow under your left shoulder and your left hand under your head.

Finally, squeeze the nipple of each breast between your thumb and index finger; be gentle, but squeeze firmly enough to perform an adequate test. If there is any discharge whatsoever from the nipple—either clear or bloody—report it to your doctor immediately. (An exception, of course, would be milk in a nursing mother.)

If you or your doctor determines that you are a high-risk individual who is more prone than others to develop breast cancer, your doctor will probably want to give you more sophisticated tests regularly that detect cancer before either you or the doctor could feel a lump or thickening.

Probably the most common form of early detection is by *mammography*—examination of the breast by X ray. Recent advances in science have refined this method (through the use of special tubes, filters, and films) so that only a minute amount of radiation is used in the examination, thus reducing the risk of exposing you to too much radiation (a cancer-causing agent itself!). Authorities agree that because of the highly refined equipment you run no risk of developing cancer as a result of mammography examinations, even if you have a number of them over a number of years. (Even if you are not a high-risk individual, some doctors are now recommending this exam for every woman once a year.)

There are two views taken of your breast: one is an up-and-down view (called a cranio-caudad), and the other is a side-to-side view (called a medio-lateral). The examination, of course, is painless; the dual view permits the complete breast to be examined.

The second method of early detection is called *thermography*—a method that uses no X ray but that depends on a device called a thermograph. The test is quick and painless. Because cancerous growths emit certain heat patterns, the sensitive thermograph is placed next to the breast; it records and picks up heat transmitted from the breast and records that pattern into a photographic image. Your doctor can then tell if anything unusual is going on.

How often should you be examined by a doctor? Every woman over the age of thirty-five should have a thorough, complete breast examination by a doctor once a year. Some women should have physician examinations twice a year: women who have had a mastectomy; women who have had a number of breast surgeries or who have had their breasts injured in accidents (rendering conventional examination difficult because of the amount of scar tissue); women who have shown large masses on a mammography; women whose thermography exams indicate abnormalities; and women whose family history reveals two or more close relatives with breast cancer. These women should have biannual examinations regardless of age.

Treatment of breast cancer includes surgery (mastectomy, either simple or radical, may be used) and hormonal treatment.

What can you do to protect yourself against breast cancer? Your hands are your best weapons. Use them. And learn whether you are a high-risk woman; if you are, confer with your physician and arrange for appropriate tests. Factors that determine high risk include:[20]

Sex. Ninety-nine percent of all breast cancers occur in women.

82

Age. Seventy-five percent of all breast cancers occur in women over the age of forty.

Family history. Especially in a mother, sister, or aunt.

Bearing children. Women who are unmarried or infertile, women with less than three children, and women who had their first child after the age of thirty-four run a substantially higher risk.

Previous cancer in one breast. There is a five times greater than normal chance that cancer will develop in the other breast, too.

Disease. Certain diseases—among them precancerous mastopathy—increase the predisposition to breast cancer.

Prolonged menstruation. Women who menstruate for thirty or more years run an increased risk; so do women who begin menstruating before they are twelve or who do not stop menstruating until they are over thirty-five. Women who complete menopause before they are thirty-seven (even if it is artificial) have much less chance of developing breast cancer.

Cancer elsewhere in the body. There is a 30-percent greater chance of your developing breast cancer if you have had cancer of another organ—the ovary, colon, endometrium, or salivary gland, especially.

Wet earwax. For some reason, women who are genetically prone to develop breast cancer also produce wet—not dry and flaky—earwax.

High fat intake. You run a significantly high risk if your diet is rich in fat.

Obesity. You are much more prone to develop breast cancer if you are obese—first, because your diet is probably higher in fat, and second, because obesity tends to stimulate production of certain kinds of hormones that may trigger dormant cancer cells into activity.

Diabetes, hypertension, and/or hypothyroidism.

Chronic psychological stress. Women who are under constant psychological stress tend to produce corticosteroids, which interfere with the body's natural immunity processes and which can foster cancer.

83

Exposure to heavy doses of radiation. However, mammography does not produce sufficient amounts of radiation to be harmful, even considering cumulative effects.

Organ transplant. The drugs required by a transplant patient that prevent the patient from rejecting the organ tend to suppress the body's natural immunity systems, much as do the corticosteroids produced by stress.

Viruses in mother's milk. Because certain viruses can be transmitted to an infant through the mother's milk, women with a family history of breast cancer should not breast-feed their children; the virus might be transmitted before the cancer is ever discovered or diagnosed.

Hormone imbalance.

Estrogen administration. While researchers do not know whether medications containing estrogen *cause* cancer, they do think that these estrogen substances can stimulate cancers that already exist to develop more rapidly and can stimulate dormant or inactive cancers to become activated.

COLON AND RECTUM

About 102,000 people in the United States each year develop cancer of the colon and/or rectum; about half of them die.[21] More people in the United States have cancer of the colon and/or rectum than any other kind of cancer. Again, early diagnosis is critical: Cancer of the colon and/or rectum is considered highly curable if it is found in time—before it spreads to another part of the body.

Major symptoms of cancer of the colon and/or rectum include a change in the bowel habits and bleeding in the stools. If you notice either of these, contact your physician immediately—especially if you are a high-risk individual. Specific risk factors will be identified later in this chapter.

Again, it is important to understand a little about the structure of the colon and rectum before you can understand the cancer that affects them. The colon (sometimes called the large bowel) is the last five to six feet of the large intestine; the rectum, composing the last five or six inches of the colon, leads to the outside of the body. The solid and semisolid wastes from the digestive tract are eliminated through the colon and rectum. Symptoms lasting longer than two weeks (including constipation, diarrhea, abdominal discomfort or pain, or blood in the stool, either bright red or black) are signals that you should check with a doctor immediately.

Many cancers in the colon start out as *polyps*—pendulous little growths that extend from the intestinal wall. Some people have a hereditary condition where the polyps are clustered together in large beds; a great percentage of the time, these develop into cancers. Individual polyps, however, are usually benign, and most stay that way.[22]

However, when these cherrylike polyps are not removed—even the individual ones—they can lead to cancer over a period of time due to the irritation present in the bowel as wastes are eliminated from the body.[23]

Diagnosis, as discussed in more detail later in the chapter, consists of examination by a doctor with a sigmoidoscope, an instrument that allows the doctor to see clearly the lower ten to twelve inches of the colon. If the doctor sees a small growth or polyp or any unusual tissue, he or she can remove it through the sigmoidoscope; it can then be sent to a laboratory for a biopsy.

Other diagnostic procedures include X ray (including a barium enema), tests for blood in the stool, and tests with a colonoscope—an instrument no bigger around than your finger, so highly flexible that it can be maneuvered through the entire colon. The colonoscope emits brilliant rays of light that enable the physician to see the lining of the colon clearly.

Treatments for cancer of the colon or rectum depend on the severity and location of the cancer. If the physician finds that you have a polyp, he can probably remove it easily and safely in his office. If the polyp is benign, you will require no further treatment but will probably be asked to have extensive examinations more regularly to check for the possible growth of other polyps that might eventually lead to cancer.

If your doctor finds a malignant tumor or polyp, your treatment will depend on your age, your medical history, your general health, and the type and location of your cancer. Surgery is almost always used in the treatment of malignant growth in the colon or rectum.

If the cancer is in your rectum, you will probably need a colostomy—a surgical opening of the bowel that connects part of the colon to the outside abdominal wall, giving you a new (and a substitute) rectum. Body wastes are eliminated through this new opening into a bag that is specially designed for the purpose and that you will have to empty as needed. If your rectum is surgically removed, the colostomy will be permanent; if a large portion of the colon is removed, the colostomy will also be permanent. If a small portion of the colon is removed or if the rectum is simply operated on but not removed, your colostomy will be temporary: You will have it as long as it takes your colon and/or rectum to heal sufficiently to function again in the role of elimination of waste matter. Many people are frightened of the prospect of a colostomy, but it is a way to maintain bowel function, permitting you to lead an otherwise normal and productive life.

Other treatment options include chemotherapy, radiation therapy, or a combination that includes surgery.

LUNG

One of the most dismal forms of cancer, lung cancer claims about 90 percent of its victims; about 99,000 new cases are reported each year in the United States alone.

Symptoms include a persistent cough or any other kind of lingering respiratory ailment. Of course, it is natural for a cold to be accompanied by a cough, but any cough or respiratory ailment that lasts longer than two weeks should signal you to contact a doctor.

Researchers have been able to isolate the causes of lung cancer much better than they have been able to isolate the causes of many other kinds of cancer; some estimate that if no one smoked cigarettes, 80 percent of lung cancer cases would be eliminated.[24] Other causes include general pollutants, insecticides, and certain occupational hazards (as outlined later in this chapter).

Cancer of the lung is the leading cause of death among men and is a cause of rising mortality among women. About 280 people a day die from lung cancer in the United States.[25]

The best protection against cancer of the lung is to refrain from smoking. If you already smoke, stop; if there is no disease present when you stop, the body will repair any damage that has been done and you will run a significantly low risk of developing cancer of the lung.

SKIN

Skin cancer is the most common and most curable of all forms of cancer. (The exception to this is malignant melanoma, a form of cancer involving moles.) Still, about 5,000 a year die from skin cancer in the United States—a figure that is much too high, since effective treatment is so available and since cancer of the skin is so easily detected.

Each year in the United States about 120,000 people develop skin cancer, evidenced by a dry, scaly patch of skin, a tender red spot that won't heal, a mole that changes color, or an area of unusual coloring.[26]

Because it can be seen, skin cancer can almost always be detected and treated at an early stage—enabling you to prevent disfigurement and death. But, even more important, skin cancer can be *prevented*. It is up to you to learn how to prevent skin cancer and to do everything you can to protect yourself against it.

The most common skin cancers are named for the cells that are involved: basal and squamous.[27] Basal cells, composing the outermost layer of skin, produce more cancers than do squamous cells, which are located deeper and which make up most of the skin. Basal cell cancers are pale, waxy, pearly nodules or red, scaly, sharply outlined patches of skin. Cancers appearing in the squamous cells are usually scaly patches and nodules. Either kind may eventually ulcerate and form crusts.

A less common—but much more dangerous—form of skin cancer is melanoma. Melanomas are usually black or dark brown; in occasional victims they lack pigmentation altogether. They resemble moles; some even arise from moles. Often a melanoma will ulcerate and bleed easily if it is irritated or slightly injured.

Metastasis is the most critical danger of skin cancer: Most skin cancers that are left untreated spread to involve other organs of the body, which can result in more complex cancers and, eventually, death. Basal cell cancers rarely metastasize; squamous cell cancers usually do. Though few basal or squamous cell cancers result in death, almost half of all cases of melanoma claim their victims.[28]

What is the leading cause of skin cancer? The sun. The ultraviolet rays in sunlight—the ones that cause you to tan and burn—are the same ones that cause cancer in basal and squamous cells. Almost all skin cancers are caused by the sun, but some are a result of aging, heredity, tar, arsenic, X rays, heat, or other disease elsewhere in the body (including metastasis from other cancers).[29]

Anyone can develop skin cancer, but you run a greater risk if you have red hair and a fair complexion; people tend to inherit the *susceptibility* to the disease, but not the cancer itself.[30] Complexion and coloring don't completely determine risk of developing the disease, though: Even blacks can develop skin cancer.

The ultraviolet rays of the sun—the ones that cause the cancer—easily penetrate through clouds, so indirect sunlight can expose you to as great a risk as can direct, intense sunlight. And, of course, prolonged exposure greatly increases your risk of developing skin cancer.

What can you do to protect yourself against developing skin cancer? First, report to your doctor *immediately* if you notice a persistent skin ulcer, a persistent scaly patch, a mole that gets bigger or bleeds or gets darker, or a firm sore that will not heal or that increases in size. Early detection is on your side; some researchers claim that as many as 100 percent of all skin cancers could be cured if they were detected early in the course of the disease.

If you have to be in the sun, take some or all of the following precautions:[31]

Try to tan instead of burn; start your exposure to the sun slowly, and gradually build up your exposure time.

Keep covered up if you must be in the sun for a long period of time. Avoid gauze fabrics or lightweight, loosely knit fabrics; white shirts, for instance, provide almost no protection. Wear dark colors and tightly weaved clothing; wear a hat, and make sure your shirt is long-sleeved. Cover as much skin as you can.

If your hair is long, leave it down over your ears and neck instead of braiding or styling it on top of your head. Hair—even light blond hair—is an excellent protection against the sun's rays.

Use a strong sunscreen, preferably one listing para-aminobenzoic acid (PABA) as an ingredient. Make sure that you apply it after swimming or showering and that you reapply it every time you are in water that might wash it from your skin (including heavy perspiration). Also make sure that you apply it liberally to *all* of your skin—even skin that will be covered by clothing.

If you can, stay in the shade.

If you can, stay out of the sun at midday. The hour on either side of noon will expose you to fully a third of the day's ultraviolet rays.

Assess what around you might be reflecting the sun's rays. Sand is one of the worst offenders: A beach umbrella, which often provides a false sense of security, actually serves instead to trap the sun's rays underneath the umbrella, where you are sitting.

There are other things you can do to protect yourself from developing skin cancer:

Avoid contact with the sun if you are taking medication that may increase your photosensitivity and reaction to the sun's rays. Medication taken for urinary tract infection (sulfonamides), mild diabetes (hypoglycemics taken orally), high blood pressure (diuretics), anxiety (tranquilizers), allergies (antihistamines), acne and frequent infection (tetracycline), fungal infections, psoriasis, obesity (saccharin and other artificial sweeteners), and some psychological problems (chlordiazepoxide hydrochloride) can make you extremely sensitive to the sun. Other common items that will increase your reaction include antiseptic soaps, quinine used in soft drinks and mixers, and fragrances used in soaps, perfumes, and cosmetics.

If you are forced to be in the sun for long periods of time, wear gloves: Many skin cancers start on the hands because they are so rarely covered or protected.

Inspect your body carefully and regularly. Use a full-length mirror, and use a hand mirror so that you can inspect your back and buttocks. See your doctor immediately if a mole changes size or color, if a lump develops, or if a blemish or mark on your skin bleeds or changes color.

Those four cancers—breast, colon/rectum, lung, and skin—are the most common and claim the most lives in the United States each year. The eight other most common—oral, uterus, kidney and bladder, larynx, prostate, stomach, leukemia, and lymph—can be detected if you subject yourself to regular and thorough physical examinations and if you alert your doctor as soon as you recognize one of the seven warning signals of cancer (any of the following that last more than a week):

1. A change in bowel or bladder habits.
2. A sore that does not heal.
3. Unusual bleeding or discharge.
4. Thickening or lump in the breast or elsewhere.

5. Indigestion or difficulty in swallowing.

6. Obvious change in a wart or mole.

7. Nagging cough or hoarseness.

HIGH-RISK INDIVIDUALS

Four factors tend to signal high risk for cancer in general: overweight, smoking, drinking alcoholic beverages, and development of cancer in an immediate member of one's family. According to the American Cancer Society, certain factors indicate high risk for certain kinds of cancer:[32]

LUNG
1. The person is a heavy smoker who is over the age of fifty.
2. The person has smoked a pack of cigarettes a day for twenty years.
3. The person has developed a "smoker's hack."
4. The person started smoking at or before the age of fifteen.
5. The smoker is working with or near asbestos.

BREAST
1. The person detects a lump in the breast.
2. The person suffers nipple discharge.
3. The person has close relatives who have developed breast cancer.
4. The person is over the age of thirty-five; the risk increases if the person is over the age of fifty.
5. The woman has never had children or had her first child after she was thirty years old.

COLON/RECTUM
1. The person has had rectal polyps.
2. Rectal polyps run in the person's family.
3. The person has suffered from ulcerative colitis at some time in his or her life.
4. The person has had blood in the stools.
5. The person is over the age of forty.

UTERUS/CERVIX
1. The woman has suffered from unusual bleeding or discharge.
2. The woman had frequent sexual relations in her early teens.
3. The woman has had many sexual partners.
4. The woman comes from a low-income background.
5. The woman had poor medical care during or following a pregnancy.
6. The woman is between the ages of forty and forty-nine.

UTERUS/ENDOMETRIUM
1. The woman has suffered from unusual bleeding or discharge.
2. The woman undergoes menopause after she is fifty-five.
3. The woman has diabetes.
4. The woman has high blood pressure.
5. The woman is overweight.
6. The woman is between the ages of fifty and sixty-four.

SKIN
1. The person has excessive exposure to the sun.
2. The person is fair-complected.
3. The person works with coal tar, pitch, or creosote.

ORAL
1. The person smokes heavily.
2. The person drinks heavily.
3. The person has poor oral hygiene.

OVARY
1. The woman has a family history of ovarian cancer.
2. The woman is between the ages of fifty and fifty-nine.

PROSTATE
1. The man is over the age of sixty-five.
2. The man experiences difficulty in urinating.

STOMACH
1. The person consumes a diet heavy in salted, smoked, or pickled foods.
2. The person has some link with the ''A'' blood group.
3. The person comes from a family with a history of stomach cancer.

There are a number of additional factors associated with high or low cancer risks:[33]

Heredity. While there is no conclusive proof, evidence suggests that there is a definite tendency of familial patterns of risk in cancers of the breast (female only), stomach, large intestine, endometrium, prostate, lung, and ovary. These familial patterns could be due to genetic inheritance or to environmental factors (such as diet or occupation) that remain the same from generation to generation.

Some information now available suggests that certain combinations of cancer occur in some families. For instance, some families suffer recurrent combinations of colon, stomach, and endometrium cancers; breast and ovary cancers; or brain cancer and sarcomas.

Brain tumors occur more frequently than expected in brothers and sisters of children with brain tumors. If an identical twin develops childhood leukemia, the other twin will probably develop the disease within one to two years. Some cancers—especially of the eye and thyroid—have been definitely linked to genetic mutation. And some precancerous conditions—conditions that lead to cancer—have shown marked hereditary patterns. Those include polyps in the colon and rectum, abnormal skin pigmentation, and albino characteristics.

Some relationship has been shown that links chromosome makeup with the chances of developing cancer. Persons with mongolism (Down's syndrome) have a high risk of developing leukemia, possibly due to the extra chromosome. Many individuals who have developed chronic myeloid leukemia have part of one chromosome missing (called the Philadelphia chromosome). There have even been some connections made between certain blood type groups and certain kinds of cancer.

Previous cancer. The number of individuals who develop a second primary tumor is very small in comparison with the number who develop one primary tumor, but many people develop secondary tumors or cancer sites due to metastases from the primary tumor site.

In addition, good evidence indicates that tumors occur with very high frequency in certain pairs of sites, including breast and endometrium; breast and ovary; endometrium and ovary; colon and endometrium; colon and breast; cervix and rectum; cervix and urinary bladder; rectum and urinary bladder; salivary glands and breast; lip and skin; and upper digestive and respiratory systems.

In a few instances cancer of a certain site carries with it a very high risk of developing a second cancer in the same organ. Those organs include the skin, oral cavity, rectum, and large intestine. In other cases there is a high risk of developing a cancer in a paired organ: the opposite breast, the opposite ovary, or the opposite lung—probably due to the same factors that precipitated growth of the first cancer.

Marital status. As with most causes of death (and in most countries), married persons are less likely to die from cancer than are single persons. There might be several reasons for this: Persons who are in poor health generally are frequently not chosen as marriage partners, or are less likely to remarry, and are thus more likely to die single. The statistics may also be due to the fact that marital status might erroneously be left off death certificates.

The differences in marital status for men is pretty marked; with women, it doesn't make much difference except in cases of breast or genital cancer (especially cervical cancer). Women who develop breast cancer are much more likely to be single; those developing cancer of the reproductive organs are much more likely to be married and to have had their first child at a late age.

Socioeconomic status. Studies made of groups in the United States and Western Europe indicate that people in lower socioeconomic groups had an above-average incidence and death rate from all kinds of cancer. This is especially true in cases of cancer of the cervix, esophagus, and stomach; the lowest economic group had the highest incidence of lung cancer. On the other hand, the low economic groups also had a low incidence of breast cancer in females.

Economic status as an indicator of cancer risk is not fully understood; lower-income persons may develop more cancer because of their general lifestyle, their lack of quality medical care, and their exposure to cancer-causing agents in the environment.

Social customs. Most social customs and living habits that increase risk of developing cancer originate in Oriental and Asian countries. For instance, chewing betel (common in Southeast Asia) contributes heavily to cancer of the oral cavity; in India the same cancer is caused by chewing khaini (a combination of tobacco and lime).

Skin cancer is caused by keeping heated pots next to the abdomen (common in Kashmir and Japan), by wearing loin cloths (common in India), and by sitting on a heated brick platform (common in China). Countries that discourage circumcision develop high rates of cancer of the penis.

Cigarette smoking. According to detailed and comprehensive studies, cigarette smoking is the main cause of lung cancer among men; the studies show that the risk of developing lung cancer increases with the number of cigarettes smoked per day and the duration of the smoking habit; the risk is greater, the earlier the age at which smoking was started. These studies also show that the risk of developing lung cancer lessens after a person stops smoking.

Cigarette smoking also causes lung cancer among women, but there are fewer cases—probably due to the fact that women generally smoke fewer cigarettes, generally smoke low-tar and filtered cigarettes more frequently than do men, and generally inhale lower levels of smoke.

Smoking pipes or cigars causes less lung cancer than does smoking cigarettes, but pipe and cigar smoking causes more lip and oral cancer than does cigarette smoking.

Smokers who suffer from chronic bronchitis suffer an exceptionally high risk of developing lung cancer—and that risk is often independent of age or number of cigarettes consumed. Lung cancer deaths are also greater among urban populations—probably because of occupational hazards encountered in urban areas.

Cigarette smoking also increases the risk of developing cancer in sites other than the lungs. Cigarette smoking has been definitely linked to cancer of the larynx, the oral cavity, the urinary bladder, and the lip.

Diet. Some organic chemicals used in food processing have caused cancer in animals; these include dyes and synthetic flavorings. Another very possible carcinogen is the estrogen preparation used to fatten and tenderize animals prior to slaughter and consumption.

Certain dietary deficiencies may also contribute to risk of cancer. Multiple dietary deficiencies may cause cancer of the oropharynx and esophagus; iodine deficiency probably causes or contributes heavily to cancer of the thyroid. Malnourishment is a huge factor in development of cancer of the liver.

The amount of bulk in the diet may also be significant: Among populations regularly consuming diets high in bulk (such as the Oriental populations), cancer of the colon is much lower than among those populations (in North America and Western Europe) that consume highly refined foods rich in starch and low in bulk.

There is also an indirect link to diet: Obese men and women are much more likely to develop cancer, especially of the endometrium, pancreas, gallbladder, and breast.

Alcohol consumption. Alcohol consumption increases the risk of developing cancer of the buccal cavity, pharynx, larynx, and esophagus. This is due to two factors: There are suspected carcinogens in the alcohol (a result of distilling and fermentation), and persons who consume large quantities of alcohol tend to eat improperly and suffer from malnutrition, which is a precursor of several forms of cancer.

Exposure to radiation. Because of the increasing use of radioactive substances in industry and medicine and because of tests of nuclear weapons (and the subsequent fallout), radiation-caused cancers will probably increase significantly during the next few years. Until now, most of these cancers have been related to X rays used for medical purposes and to radioactive isotopes in the environment.

Radiation causes several kinds of cancers, depending on the kind of radiation and the kind of exposure. Radium workers develop skin cancers and leukemia; radium-dial painters develop bone cancer; X-ray technicians who do not take proper precautions to protect themselves develop excessively high rates of leukemia. Uranium mine workers develop lung cancer; survivors of the atomic bomb attacks on Hiroshima and Nagasaki have suffered unusually high leukemia death rates, especially in the first ten years following the explosion.

Sometimes patients treated with radiotherapy for other illnesses develop cancer as a result of the X-ray treatments. For years children were treated with X rays of the neck to reduce enlargements of the thymus glands; the result was an increase in cancer of the thyroid. Irradiation of the spine used in some medical treatments was found to cause cancer of the lung and leukemia. Exposure of pregnant women to X rays has been found to cause increased rates of leukemia and other malignancies in their children.

Occupation. Because of environmental risks, members of certain occupations develop certain cancers at an abnormally high rate. Those whose occupations expose them to certain substances run an increased risk of developing certain cancers, including arsenic (skin, lung); coal tar, pitch (skin, lung); petroleum (skin, lung); shale oils (skin); lignite tar and paraffin (skin); creosote oils (skin); anthracene oils (skin); soot carbon black (skin); mustard gas (lung); mineral oils (skin, respiratory, and upper alimentary tracts); coal carbonization products (lung, bladder); sunlight (skin); chromates (lung); asbestos (lung, pleura, peritoneum, gastrointestinal tract); aromatic amines, dyes, and rubber (bladder, biliary tract, and salivary glands); X rays (skin, lung, leukemia); nickel (lung, nasal cavity, and sinus); benzol (leukemia); isopropyl oil (lung, larynx, and nasal sinus); wood furniture working (nasal cavity, sinus); leather working (nasal cavity, sinus, and bladder); and soft coal mining (stomach).

Other disease. Certain other diseases increase your risk of developing cancer. White patches of the mouth (leukoplakia) often precede cancer of the mouth; chronic bone diseases often precede bone cancer.

Polyps of the rectum and colon (found in ulcerative colitis and familial polyposis) usually indicate a high susceptibility to cancer of the colon. Polyps in the stomach and endometrium also signal the onset of cancer.

Those with diabetes run a high risk of developing cancer of the pancreas and increase the risk of developing a number of other cancers. Short-term infections rarely cause cancer; long-term infections often do. Certain disorders of the immunity system often cause cancer of the lymph system. Patients who are given drug therapy to prevent rejection of an implanted organ develop cancer at extremely high rates.

Individuals who suffer from cirrhosis of the liver often develop cancer of the liver, especially in underdeveloped countries. Cancer also appears rapidly following severe emotional strain or mental illness; researchers can find no explanation and no definite link.

Certain congenital defects—among them Down's syndrome, Bloom's syndrome, Fanconi's syndrome, and certain immunologic disorders—also cause certain cancers.

In some cases, however, presence of a certain disease seems to offer almost a protection against cancer. Extremely low rates have been associated with tuberculosis, atherosclerosis, and hypertension.

Benign disease. Benign diseases do not turn into cancer, but the presence of a benign disease increases your risk of developing cancer because the same conditions that led to development of the benign disease may become more pronounced and lead to a malignant disease, or cancer. For instance, leukoplakia —white patches on the mucous membranes of the mouth—is caused by a combination of malnutrition, local irritation, and poor dental and oral hygiene. When these factors become severe, cancer of the mouth often develops. The leukoplakia did not cause the cancer, nor did it turn into cancer; the conditions that caused the leukoplakia went uncorrected, became more severe, and led to development of mouth cancer.

DIAGNOSING CANCER

Diagnosing cancer often involves a complex network of laboratory tests designed to give physicians a clear picture of cellular activity in any suspected cancer area. But before any diagnostic tests take place, two simple things occur: You recognize that you may have cancer (either because you have recognized one of cancer's seven warning signals or because you know that you are a high-risk individual), and your doctor performs a thorough physical examination to confirm that there may be a problem and that you need further testing.

The most important key to combating cancer is early detection. What does this mean to you? You should honestly assess your risk rate. If you know that you have a tendency toward a certain kind of cancer, or if you have been exposed to definite carcinogens, inform your physician so that he can be on the alert. Many kinds of cancer can be diagnosed *before symptoms even occur* if patients and doctors work together in assessing risks and keeping an eye on potential trouble spots.

But, eventually, in most kinds of cancer symptoms will appear. It is *critical* that you learn the seven warning signs of cancer (listed earlier in this chapter) and that you report to your physician *immediately* if one or more of the symptoms persist for more than a week. Then, depending on your own particular set of symptoms, your doctor will examine you and possibly recommend further tests.

In certain kinds of cancer there are tests you can perform yourself on a regular basis that will help you discover any potential problems as early as possible. You should conduct these tests on yourself once each month; after reading these general instructions, ask your doctor to help instruct you if you have any further questions.

ORAL/FACIAL CANCER

Most people are aware of the importance of breast self-examination, but few know that regular oral/facial examination is as simple and even more critical: Oral/facial cancers occur at about four times the rate of breast cancers.[34]

All you need to perform the examination is a well-lighted mirror, a gauze pad or handkerchief (clean, of course), and your own index finger—well washed. Examine these areas in the following ways:

Face. Look at the skin of your face, neck, and lips. See if any of the skin has changed color without explanation and see if you have any lumps or sores. Make sure you look at the area that is usually covered by your eyeglasses if you wear them.

Outer cheeks. Feel your outer cheeks carefully. Are there any lumps or swellings? Do you feel tenderness? Feel them all the way back to your ears and all the way down to your jaw.

Neck. Feel your neck closely, all the way around, paying special attention to the sides, where the lymph glands lie, and to your Adam's apple area. Is there tenderness, or do you feel lumps?

Roof of the mouth. Tilt your head back, and use your well-lighted mirror to look at both your hard and soft palates. Note any abnormalities in coloring, tenderness, growths, and so on.

Tongue. You need to look at both the topside and underside of your tongue, again with the well-lighted mirror. Grasp your tongue with the gauze or handkerchief, and pull it out; extend it in all directions so that you get a good look at it from all sides. Note any growths, sores, or ulcerated areas.

Inner cheek. Use your index finger on the inside and your thumb on the outside to expose the lining of your cheek. Look for any ulcerations, growths, or white, red, or dark patches.

Lips. Evert your upper lip, and look for any possible white, red, or dark patches. Do the same with your lower lip. Also check for growths or sores.

Floor of the mouth. Lift up your tongue, and examine the floor of your mouth that is located underneath your tongue. If you've never looked under your tongue before, you will find a rainbow of colors and a whole bevy of lumps. It's a good idea to have your doctor or dentist point out during your next examination what is normal, and what you should be looking for.

You should perform this self-examination more often if you drink or smoke. If you smoke a pipe, pay special attention to your lips during regular checks.

SKIN CANCER

Look carefully at your skin, as described earlier in this chapter, using a full-length mirror and a hand mirror to examine your back and buttocks. Look for any unexplained changes in pigmentation, coloring, or texture. Watch for sores or ulcerations of any kind, and note any dry, scaly areas. Briefly feel your skin, searching for lumps, swelling, or other conditions that might signal a problem.

BREAST CANCER

Using the instructions listed earlier in this chapter for breast self-examination, note any irregular contours, skin dimpling, thickening of tissue, lumps, or hard masses. Check the lymph nodes in your armpits to detect any swelling or tenderness.

A number of highly refined tests are available to physicians who are trained in testing procedures. Depending on your individual case, your doctor will decide which tests and diagnostic procedures are best and most reliable.

CANCER TREATMENT

Treatment for cancer, of course, depends on the kind of cancer, where it is located, the patient's general health, and the patient's medical history. There are currently only three general methods for controlling or eliminating cancer: surgical removal of cancerous tissue, radiation therapy, and chemotherapy. These can be varied and combined in a number of ways, but they remain the only approved methods.

Unfortunately, cancer victims are increasingly also becoming victims of cancer quacks: doctors who prescribe unorthodox—and ineffective—methods of treatment at skyrocketing costs, promising cure to people who don't know any better. According to recent estimates, about one-third of all people who are diagnosed as having cancer comply with their doctors' suggestions and treatments. The other two-thirds eventually are "treated" by quacks.

Why?

People of all ages, socio-economic classes, educational levels, ethnic backgrounds, and geographic areas seek the services of quacks for many different reasons.

Probably the primary motivation for turning to quacks is fear. Cancer is certainly a disease that strikes fear—especially fear of death—in its victims. The fear of death can cause one to seek help anywhere. Many victims may also fear orthodox medical treatments such as surgery, which could result in disfigurement or pain.

Others go to quacks through simple ignorance. They are not able to distinguish between legitimate and unorthodox medical care and practitioners.

Since cancer treatment is not a simple or short process, many become weary of the time, pain, discomfort, or complexity involved and, therefore turn in frustration or impatience to someone who promises a quick or simple cure—something that only a quack can provide.

Many seek miracle cures. Often valuable time and money are spent on the hope for a miracle from treatments that involve more faith than practical efforts. As an example, Helene Brown of the American Cancer Society (California Division) offers the case of a woman who relies on a prayer cloth when she suspects she has breast cancer. She faithfully depends on the powers of this prayer cloth to shrink the growing mass. After six months of dependence on this hope, she consults a doctor and finds that she does indeed have breast cancer, but also learns that the disease has progressed to an untreatable and terminal stage.[35]

And then there are those who have nowhere else to turn. After having tried everything that the medical profession has to offer, a patient may be told that nothing can be done because of the severity of the case. Such a person may not want to face the terminal nature of the cancer and the probability of death in a matter of weeks or months and may reach out in a last attempt at anything. When the medical profession can do no more, the victim may turn to a quack who will usually offer some kind of positive reassurance, but little in the way of actual treatment or results.

It is tragic to realize that most people who turn to quacks have cancers that are still in early, curable stages. The time a patient spends with the quack simply allows the cancer to grow larger, out of control—to spread to other organs in the body, until there is really no chance for cure. But there's another tragic aspect, too: There are a number of people who go to cancer quacks who don't have cancer at all; they're just afraid that they have cancer. Unfortunately, most of these unscrupulous "doctors" have no conscience when it comes to taking a victim's money. They'll keep you believing that you have cancer and that you are getting cured as long as you keep handing over the money.

How can you tell which is a quack and which is a legitimate doctor? Mere appearance isn't the key: Quacks are usually well-dressed, neat, and friendly; they greet you with warmth and reassurance. Some are even licensed MDs; their offices come complete with white-uniformed nurses, fancy equipment, and comfortable waiting rooms. The American Cancer Society has outlined several clues that will help you determine which is which:

The quack claims to have a "secret" cure for cancer and often offers treatment you can only get from his or her clinic. The treatment sometimes bears the doctor's own name. The quack will tell you that he or she is being sabotaged by members of the medical profession (perhaps because they are jealous of his cure) but will willingly show you letters of testimonial from patients who have been cured. You are discouraged from going to another doctor for a second opinion and discouraged from checking with any medical specialists about your treatment.

A reputable doctor does not offer "exclusive" treatments. The treatments he or she prescribes are generally and widely available from other doctors and in many hospitals. The doctor's membership in professional medical associations (such as the AMA) is a matter of public record. You are not offered a patented treatment, and your treatment does not bear the doctor's own name or the name of his or her firm. The doctor will refuse to divulge the details of other patients' cases to you or to any members of the public; he or she respects a patient's confidentiality and right to privacy. The doctor will refuse to treat you for cancer until cancer has been definitely confirmed by laboratory tests, and he or she insists on making a final diagnosis—with the help of other doctors if necessary —before initiating treatment. The doctor *always* welcomes advice and consultation from colleagues, and he or she will encourage you to seek a second opinion if you want one.

PREVENTING CANCER

There are many things you can do to reduce your risk of getting cancer; some estimate that up to 50 percent—or half—of all cancer cases are preventable.* Some prevention techniques have been discussed earlier in the chapter, but a brief summary would include the following practices:

Eat less high-fat beef, lamb, and pork; instead, eat more fish and poultry. Further cut back on fat by choosing leaner cuts of red meat—flank, round, and rump—when you can, and trim all visible fat off meat before cooking. Use

*This section adapted and summarized from Jane E. Brody, "A Way to Reduce Your Chances of Getting Cancer," *Reader's Digest,* November 1977, pp. 131–34; Ruth Winter, "10 Ways You Can Avoid Cancer," *Science Digest,* May 1973, pp. 33–37; Guy R. Newell and Norma Golumbic, "What You Can Do to Protect Yourself Against Cancer," *AORN Journal,* 25, no. 5 (April 1977) 909–22; Nicholas Gonzalez, "Preventing Cancer," *Family Health/Today's Health,* May 1976, pp. 30–34, 69–74.

lowfat or nonfat milk in place of regular whole milk, and choose dairy products that are processed with lowfat or nonfat milk. Use polyunsaturated margarines in place of such table fats as butter.

Bake, broil, roast, or stew food instead of frying or deep-frying food. When you cook a stew or soup, make it ahead of time, refrigerate it overnight, and remove all the fat that has congealed before you rewarm and eat the food.

Eat no more than two to three eggs a week.

Use only liquid vegetable oils; corn or soybean oil is best. Never use solid shortenings in cooking.

Avoid sugar as much as possible. Don't add sugar at the table; go easy on candy, pies, cakes, pastries, cookies, sweet rolls, and other sweetened foods. Buy cereal that is not sweetened; buy fruit canned in its own juice or in light syrup, not heavy syrup. Check ingredient labels on food, and avoid those that list sugar, glucose, sucrose, fructose, corn syrup, or artificial sweeteners high in the ingredients list. (If sugar is listed first, it means that there is more sugar than anything else in that food!)

Eat more vegetables, beans, whole grains, and fruits.

Don't smoke and avoid smoke-filled rooms.

Avoid contact with car fumes and factory exhaust.

Don't get X rays unless you really need them; refuse to let your doctor X ray you as a routine "just to make sure everything checks out." X rays should be used only as needed in diagnostic work, and your doctor should be able to justify the use of every X ray he prescribes.

Limit your exposure to the sun. Use strong sunscreens when you are in the sun, and make sure you reapply them after swimming, showering, or perspiring heavily.

Avoid long exposure to household solvent cleaners, cleaning fluids, and paint thinners.

Avoid eating too many smoked or pickled foods, and don't use artificial sweeteners.

Don't drink alcohol.

Take great caution when you use pesticides, fungicides, and other garden and lawn chemicals.

Choose your occupation carefully; think twice about those that place you at a high risk of developing cancer.

Be careful about contraception. If possible, avoid using oral contraceptives.

Don't take any kind of medication needlessly.

Avoid chronic infection and irritation.

When you buy bread, make sure that it contains whole grain *and* yeast. When you bake with flour, use whole-wheat and whole-grain as often as you can.

Examine your breasts once a month; conduct a thorough oral/facial and skin examination monthly (more often if you are a high-risk individual). Conduct any other self-examinations that your doctor recommends.

Have regular physical checkups.

Learn the seven warning signals of cancer, and report to your doctor immediately if one persists longer than one week.

Many kinds of cancer are unavoidable, but many others *can* be avoided. It's your responsibility—you call the shots. You have the opportunity of adopting a healthier life-style, one that will lead to conquering cancer in your lifetime.

REFERENCES

[1]*The Cancer Story* (Washington, D.C.: U.S. Department of Health, Education and Welfare, Public Health Service, National Institutes of Health, 1970), no. 77–210, p. 2.

[2] I. J. Fidler and M. L. Kripke, "Tumor Growth and Spread," *Chemistry,* 50, no. 1 (January–February 1977), 18–24.

[3]Gene Bylinsky, "Cancer Cells Begin to Yield Their Secrets," *Fortune,* November 1971, p. 156.

[4]William H. Leitch, "Review Your Knowledge of Tumors," *AORN Journal,* February 1973, p. 72.

[5]Lois Ember, "Environmental Cancers: Humans as the Experimental Model?" *Environmental Science and Technology,* 10, no. 13 (December 1976), 1190–95.

[6]"Cancer Linked to Personality Traits," *Medical World News,* May 31, 1976, pp. 17–18.

[7]"New Breed of Pollutants: The Dangers They Carry," *U.S. News and World Report,* February 7, 1977, pp. 42–46.

[8]"New Breed of Pollutants," pp. 42–43.

[9]"Cancer Hazards in the Modern Environment," *Progress Against Cancer* (Washington, D.C.: U.S. Department of Health, Education and Welfare, National Advisory Council, Public Health Service, National Institutes of Health, 1976), DHEW No. 76–1040, pp. 18–20.

[10]"Scare Over Cancer in Water—What Research Shows," *U.S. News and World Report,* December 2, 1974, p. 61.

[11]"Fluoridation: The Cancer Scare," *Consumer Reports,* July 1978, pp. 392–96.

[12]"What Causes Cancer?" *Newsweek,* January 26, 1976, pp. 62–67.

[13] "Cancer Specter: Mutagens Found in Well-Done Beef," *Medical World News,* June 12, 1978, p. 20.

[14] "Can Diet Cause Cancer?" *Current Prescribing,* January 1977, p. 35.

[15] "Predicting Cancer Occurrence," *Medical World News,* September 20, 1976.

[16] "Changing Concepts in the Management of Breast Disease," *Medical Times,* 105, no. 3 (March 1977), 50.

[17] "Fact and Fantasy About Breast Cancer," *AORN Journal,* 19, no. 4 (April 1974), 846.

[18] Information for this section is drawn from Philip Strax, M.D., *Breast Cancer is Curable* (New York: The Benjamin Company, 1974), recommended by the American Cancer Society; from Rose Kushner, "If You've Thought about Breast Cancer . . . ." (Kensington, MD.: Women's Breast Cancer Advisory Center, Inc., 1979), p. 1; and from *The Breast Cancer Digest* (Bethesda, MD.: National Cancer Institute, 1980), pp. 5–8.

[19] American Cancer Society, *How to Examine Your Breasts* (New York: American Cancer Society, May 1975).

[20] Henry P. Leis, Jr., "Risk Factors in Breast Cancer," *AORN Journal,* 22, no. 5 (November 1975), 723–29.

[21] American Cancer Society, *1978 Cancer Facts and Figures* (New York: American Cancer Society, 1977), p. 17.

[22] Clifton R. Read, "The Cancer Nobody Talks About," *Family Health,* May 1978, p. 30.

[23] *What You Need to Know About Cancer of the Colon and Rectum* (Washington, D.C.: U.S. Department of Health, Education and Welfare, Public Health Service, National Institutes of Health), publication no. (NIH) 78-1552, pp. 3–5.

[24] Third National Cancer Survey, in *1978 Cancer Facts and Figures,* p. 13.

[25] *1978 Cancer Facts and Figures,* p. 18.

[26] Clifton R. Read, "The Most Common Cancer," *Family Health,* July 1977, p. 32.

[27] Robert T. DeVore, "Sunbathing and Skin Cancer," *FDA Consumer,* May 1977, p. 15.

[28] Ibid.

[29] Robert Jackson, "Some Reminders About Skin Cancer," *Consultant,* December 1976, p. 35.

[30] Ray Hendley and John D. Burlage, "Skin Cancer: Just a Very Common Killer," *Life and Health,* March 1977, p. 30.

31Farrington Daniels, Jr., "Saving Sun Worshippers from Their 'God,' " *Medical Opinion,* July 1976, pp. 23, 27–28.

32*1978 Cancer Facts and Figures,* pp. 4–5.

33David L. Levin, Susan S. Devesa, J. David Godwin II, and Debra T. Silverman, *Cancer Rates and Risks,* 2d ed. (Washington, D.C.: U.S. Department of Health, Education and Welfare, Public Health Service, National Institutes of Health, 1974), DHEW No. 76-691, pp. 53–78.

34"Self-Exam for Orofacial Cancer," *Medical World News,* May 3, 1976, p. 23.

35Helene Brown, "Cancer Quackery: What Can You Do About It?" *Nursing 75,* May 1975, pp. 24–25.

CHRONIC
AND
COMMUNICABLE
DISEASES

The list of factors that cause disease is almost as long as the list of diseases themselves. Each disease reacts differently, and there are even differences between us as human beings that determine how a particular disease will affect each of us.

There is probably little you can do to avoid developing a chronic disorder such as arthritis, diabetes, allergy, epilepsy, or appendicitis. There *are* things you can do, though, to reduce or eliminate the adverse effects of these and other chronic diseases that you may develop during your lifetime. Prompt and aggressive treatment does much to prevent the progressive crippling of arthritis; a careful balance of diet and medication coupled with exercise can enable a diabetic to lead a normal life.

And there's plenty you can do to protect yourself against communicable disease. You have potential protection against all seven major infectious diseases, if you take advantage of immunizations; by learning the process of infection, you can learn how to adjust your environment to afford you the greatest protection against disease—and the best possible insurance of a healthy life.

CHRONIC DISEASES
ARTHRITIS

Arthritis is often called "everybody's disease" because everyone in this country is affected—directly or indirectly, physically or economically—by arthritis.[1]

The tragedy is that many people become crippled unnecessarily, and they

104

stay crippled unnecessarily; many don't understand that arthritis is seldom hopeless, and few seek and follow treatment that can either prevent disability in the first place or reduce it after it has happened.

Another tragedy is that, despite the terrible toll it exacts in both human suffering and economic waste, chronic arthritis receives bottom-of-the-pile priority for research and public action. Many tax dollars are spent to support victims who are already crippled by arthritis, but only $1.75 per victim per year is allotted by the United States government for arthritis training and research.[2] The Arthritis Foundation has sufficient funds to add only 12 cents to that figure.

If you can learn the facts about arthritis, a great deal *can* be done about arthritis; much is being done, but much more could be done.

COSTS OF ARTHRITIS

Almost everyone, if he lives long enough, will eventually develop some kind of arthritis.* It can occur at any time from infancy on; studies reveal that 97 percent of all those over the age of sixty have enough arthritis to show up on X-ray films. Currently, about 50 million Americans have arthritis to some degree; fortunately, for many of them it is slight enough that it does not cause major disability. Twenty million have arthritis severe enough to require medical care. Each year 600,000 new victims join the ranks.

As a result of research, medical costs, welfare, and lost productivity for men and women the annual cost to the national economy due to arthritis is a whopping $13 billion. The cost of human suffering in terms of pain and disability, of course, is immeasurable.

Currently, arthritis is the nation's number-one crippling disease. More than one in ten Americans has the disease, and one in four families is affected by it. Three and a half million Americans are disabled at any one time, and arthritis causes almost 15 million days of work lost annually.

DIAGNOSIS

The four major warning signs of arthritis include the following:[3]

- Persistent pain and stiffness on arising
- Pain, swelling, or tenderness in one or more joints
- Recurrence of pain, swelling, or tenderness, especially when they involve more than one joint
- Recurrent or persistent pain and stiffness in the lower back, neck, knees, and other joints

Unfortunately, aching pains in the joints or around the joints can mean a

*This section adapted from *Arthritis: The Basic Facts* (New York: Arthritis Foundation, 1976), pp. 2–3.

host of things—not just arthritis. It is critical that you be examined and diagnosed promptly if you experience any of the four warning signs of arthritis, because prompt treatment can help prevent a great deal of crippling. (For instance, some arthritis is a result of bacteria invading the joints; proper diagnosis and treatment can kill the bacteria, preventing the progression of arthritis.)

A number of diagnostic tests—including blood, urine, joint fluid, and tissue biopsy tests—may be needed to diagnose arthritis correctly, since no one test is 100-percent accurate in the diagnosis of arthritis.

RHEUMATOID ARTHRITIS

Of all the forms of arthritis, rheumatoid is the most dangerous, disabling, and destructive—and the most common.* It can strike suddenly, and it generally progresses rapidly until it reaches a seriously damaging stage.

Usually, rheumatoid arthritis strikes subtly and deceptively. The symptoms may appear for a few days and then disappear, come back a little later and disappear again, and finally return with such violence that they become a daily problem that can't be ignored. There may be days, weeks, or months between spells, and the disease may seem to go away without treatment of any kind. The pain and stiffness and swelling of joints may completely disappear, but the damage that has been done does *not* disappear. Some patients delude themselves with the idea that they have been cured, and many discontinue their treatment under such a delusion. Unfortunately, the arthritis will flare up again, often with greater intensity and disability than originally.

On the other hand, some cases are quite mild. No two cases are quite the same, and reactions vary from case to case and from month to month in the same person.

The main targets of rheumatoid arthritis are the joints of the hands and arms, the hips, the legs, and the feet, but rheumatoid arthritis sufferers are often "sick all over" because the disease attacks the connective tissues all over the body, resulting in fever, fatigue, loss of appetite, weight loss, and anemia. In many cases the lymph glands and the spleen become enlarged.

There is usually more than one joint involved in rheumatoid arthritis. Joints affected by the arthritis stiffen, then swell and become tender, eventually making full motion difficult and painful. The aching and soreness and stiffness are typically at their worst in the morning, and usually the symptoms ease up some-what after the victim has been up and moving for a while.

About a fourth of those who develop rheumatoid arthritis also develop small lumps under the skin—rheumatoid nodules—generally at the elbows.

The cause of rheumatoid arthritis is not yet known; untreated, the inflammation does progressive damage to the joints. The area where two bones meet in

---

*This and the follow six sections adapted from *Arthritis: The Basic Facts* (New York: Arthritis Foundation, 1976), pp. 7–13.

a joint is enclosed in a capsule that contains fluid. When the inner membrane of the capsule, the synovial membrane, starts to become inflamed, the membrane swells and the swelling spreads to other joint structures. Outgrowths of inflamed tissue begin eating at the cartilage surrounding the bone ends, eventually invading it and dissolving it completely. In advanced stages the scar tissue that forms between the bone ends can change to bone, and the joint becomes fused and immobile.

Rheumatoid arthritis often causes disfigurement, most readily observable in the hands, where the fingers can become drawn back and sideways.

Treatment for rheumatoid arthritis includes antiinflammatory drugs in a medication program that includes aspirin, corticosteroids, and others; a program of rest and exercise; rules of posture; splints; walking aids; and heat. In severe cases surgery and rehabilitation are used in treatment.

Risks. Some people run higher-than-average risks of developing rheumatoid arthritis. Those who have close family members—parents, grandparents, and brothers or sisters—with rheumatoid arthritis are at a higher risk of developing it than those whose close family members do not have the disease. Although rheumatoid arthritis is not hereditary, the predisposition to it is. Those who are under a great deal of emotional stress are also much more likely to develop rheumatoid arthritis; symptoms may begin after a disturbing event, and patients who already have rheumatoid arthritis find that it becomes worse after or during periods of stress.

OSTEOARTHRITIS

As common as rheumatoid arthritis, osteoarthritis is generally mild; it seldom cripples and pain is usually moderate, and almost everyone will have a touch of it if he or she lives long enough. In a few cases it can have severe results, and rarely the pain is great.

Unlike rheumatoid arthritis—which is inflammatory and which spreads from joint to joint, eventually involving the entire body—osteoarthritis confines its attack to individual joints and is rarely accompanied by inflammation.

Osteoarthritis is primarily a problem of wear and tear; the mechanical parts of the joints deteriorate with aging, and most commonly affected are the weight-bearing joints of the hips, knees, and feet. One variety that has nothing to do with the deterioration of aging or the strain on the joints occurs relatively early in life—generally during one's forties—and affects women most frequently. Heberden's nodes, bony protuberances that grow over the end joints of the fingers and toes, cause severe pain. Heberden's nodes run in families.

Osteoarthritis causes a primary change in the structure of the joints. The smooth, elastic cartilage that covers the ends of the bones becomes pitted and frayed; in some cases, the cartilage may wear away completely. As the process continues, the bone ends become thicker; bony spurs may develop, and the bone ligaments and membranes also become thickened. As the process continues, the structure of the joint is completely changed. Muscles surrounding the joint become tense and contract unnaturally as a reflex to pain; the unnatural contraction causes eventual muscle weakness.

Risks. There are likely to be several definite causes of osteoarthritis, although none has been positively identified. Researchers do know that several factors lead to a risk of developing osteoarthritis. Obesity causes more rapid degeneration of joints that bear weight, especially those of the hips, knees, and feet and ankles. Individuals who have had joints injured in accidents or in athletics are more prone to develop osteoarthritis in those joints, as are individuals who have certain joints that are exposed to unusual stress as a result of occupational or sports activities. Individuals who have hidden deformities of the joints at birth are also more likely to develop osteoarthritis later in life.

Symptoms. The major symptom of osteoarthritis is pain in and around the joints; sometimes the pain is a mild aching and soreness, and other times it is a nagging, constant pain. Because of tense muscles and muscle fatigue, the pain is occasionally felt at a distance from the joint where the trouble is.

Another major symptom is loss of ability to move a joint comfortably and easily; muscle weakness in the area surrounding the joint is common. When extreme changes in joint structure have taken place, the joints appear to be knobby from the outside.

Though there is no cure, a treatment regime of heat, drugs, rest, exercise, surgery, and rehabilitation helps prevent further damage.

JUVENILE RHEUMATOID ARTHRITIS

About 250,000 children in the United States are affected by juvenile rheumatoid arthritis, a disease similar to adult rheumatoid arthritis and an affliction that strikes girls more often than boys.

There are two major forms of juvenile rheumatoid arthritis; one erupts suddenly and violently, and the other comes on gradually. The gradual development of the second variety makes it milder; it often goes away eventually.

Skin rash, inflammation of the eyes, growth retardation, swelling of the lymph nodes and spleen, and other complications often accompany juvenile rheumatoid arthritis. In most cases proper treatment can control the disease and prevent further crippling.

GOUT

Once considered a remote affliction, gout is a form of arthritis that afflicts about 1 million Americans. Acutely painful, the disease often results from an inherited defect in body chemistry but can occur after the use of diuretic pills or medication designed to rid the body of excess fluid or to reduce blood pressure.

Uric acid, a normal chemical substance in the body, is either overproduced or produced at a rate faster than the kidneys can get rid of it; about one in ten who have excess uric acid develop gout: a condition where the uric acid forms needlelike crystals in the joints that result in severe pain and inflammation. Joints affected by gout become extremely tender, hot, and swollen.

In three out of four cases the large joint of the big toe is attacked first, but gout can settle in any joint in the body.

Risks. Researchers have isolated the following as risk factors in developing gout:[4]

- Preexisting conditions of kidney disease, rendering the kidneys incapable of totally normal functioning
- Obesity
- Injury to a joint
- Abnormal exercise, creating excess stress on joints
- Occupations that create excess stress on joints or that create excess stress on weight-bearing joints
- Consumption of alcohol, which promotes the formation of uric acid and which inhibits kidney function
- Diet low in carbohydrates, which increases the breakdown of normal tissue and which elevates the uric acid level in the blood
- Diet high in anchovies, sardines, organ meats (especially brain and liver), salmon, lentils, dried peas, and dried beans

Treatment for gout consists of medication to lower uric acid levels, to prevent overproduction of uric acid, and to ease the pain that accompanies gout.

ANKYLOSING SPONDYLITIS

Also called Marie-Strumpell disease, ankylosing spondylitis is an inflammatory disease of the spine that attacks men and women with the same frequency and that often involves other joints, especially those of the hips and shoulders.

Because small joints of the spine and the sacroiliac joints tend to be affected first, the primary symptoms are pain in the lower back and legs. Inflammation of the eyes may result as a complication, and pain may spread as the arthritis attacks other joints. As the disease progresses, the spine becomes stiff, and the stiffness continues until the spine becomes completely rigid. Curvature of the spine may eventually develop, but it can be prevented.

With proper treatment—consisting of medication, exercise, and posture routines—deformities and discomfort can be controlled. The disease usually stops of its own accord after several years; although the stiffness remains, the

109

pain is usually lessened or conquered and the victim can usually carry on a productive life.

Risks. While the definite cause is unknown, it appears that ankylosing spondylitis is a result of a hereditary predisposition; 90 percent of all those who develop the disease have a genetic marker.

SYSTEMIC LUPUS ERYTHEMATOSUS (SLE)
Systemic lupus erythematosus is a disease that inflames and may damage many tissues throughout the body. In nine out of ten cases painful arthritis is the main problem; the internal organs, joints, and skin may all be affected, and the disease often brings on symptoms that include fever, skin rash, loss of weight, weakness, fatigue, joint pain, anemia, and kidney problems.

Five times more women than men develop the disease; it most often strikes in those twenty to forty years old. While it is sometimes fatal and always serious, it can be controlled in many cases. Like rheumatoid arthritis, it follows a chronic and irregular course, and it is important for patients to stay under the guidance of a physician.

BURSITIS
The cushioning devices of the joints are called *bursa*—small sacs that contain slippery fluid and that are located at points of potential friction in the joints. Pressure or injury can cause irritation that results in inflammation of the bursa; the result is extreme tenderness and pain, and the entire joint becomes red and swollen.

Bursitis most commonly affects a shoulder, but it can occur in any joint in the body, particularly hips or elbows.

Treatment consists of pain-relieving drugs, injections of cortisone, rest, physical therapy, and, in extreme cases, surgery.

RESULTS OF INFECTION
In some cases, arthritis is directly attributable to bacteria that invade the joints and cause acute or chronic inflammation or disease. In many cases arthritis follows such bacterial diseases as tuberculosis, meningitis, and gonorrhea. Prompt diagnosis and treatment with antibiotics can completely stop the progress of the disease.[5]

COPING WITH ARTHRITIS
There are many ways you can cope with arthritis if you develop it. The most important thing to remember is *not* to attempt treatment on your own. Arthritis is a chronic disease, and proper medical treatment during all stages of the disease (even when remission is apparent) can do the most to prevent progression and crippling.

110

Arthritis is a quack's dream-come-true: It's a disease for which there is no cure (the kind that quacks thrive on), and it's painful and enduring. Watch out for quack remedies—fraudulant devices, drugs, and treatments (some of these include apple cider, vinegar, and copper wrist bracelets). Although arthritis may temporarily go into remission and the symptoms may disappear, there is currently no cure.[6]

To help cope with arthritis, try the following:

Take off extra pounds. Obesity adds stress and strain to joints and provokes and worsens arthritis. Watch your diet, though: Losing too fast can lead to gout. Also, when you have painful joints, you tend to exercise less, so your caloric consumption should be correspondingly reduced. Weight loss and loss of appetite can accompany some forms of arthritis, so it's important to eat a well-balanced diet to prevent malnutrition and anemia.

Get a sufficient amount of rest—particularly important during periods when your joints are inflamed and painful. In the past doctors recommended extensive bed rest, but experience has shown that long periods of inactivity can lead to dorformity and can have an adverse effect on circulation and muscle tone. If you have arthritis, you should plan your day's activities to include both a mid-morning and afternoon nap. You should also be sure you get enough sleep at night.

Heat is usually beneficial in relieving pain, and a warm bath first thing in the morning can help victims of arthritis get going. Specific areas of pain can benefit from hot water bottles, heating pads, or heat lamps.

Depending on the type of exercise, movement can be either good or bad for arthritis victims. Any kind of exercise that puts undue strain on the arthritic joint or that may cause inflammation should be avoided—including any kind of exercise that involves long periods of standing, lifting of heavy objects, jarring, twisting, or bending (including golf, jogging, skiing, or tennis). Most beneficial are exercises that allow the joints to move through their full range of motion without strain; swimming, especially in a heated pool, is considered to be excellent exercise for arthritis, since the joints are allowed to move in a weightless environment. Physical therapists will often provide patients with a number of individualized exercises that can gently help restore movement to arthritic joints.

Medical attention, diagnosis, and treatment should *always* be obtained and followed. Arthritis, untreated and advanced, can and does lead to death.

DIABETES

In ordinary conditions the body extracts a sugar called glucose out of foods; most glucose is derived from three basic foods, protein, carbohydrates, and fat. The glucose, or sugar, is used by the body for energy; a reserve supply is stored in various places in the body and is used as needed for reserve energy. The

111

hormone insulin, secreted into the bloodstream by the pancreas, is essential in the process of breaking down and using glucose.

In diabetes there is not enough insulin to complete this essential process. The insulin can be missing completely, can be present in insufficient supplies, or can be in a form that can't be utilized by the diabetic. The result? The glucose, a form of sugar, accumulates in the blood and stays there until the surplus can be passed through the kidneys and out of the body with the urine. As a result, the body cannot use the glucose for energy and cannot store the surplus glucose as needed for reserve energy.

There are two general kinds of diabetes: Juvenile diabetes, occurring in children, affects about 1 in 2,500 children; maturity-onset diabetes strikes 1 in 50 adults over the age of forty who did not have diabetes as children. Diabetes is one of our most common ailments; 4 million in the United States have it, another 5.5 million are potential diabetics, and over half of those who have diabetes don't know it.[7]

RISK FACTORS

Anyone can develop diabetes, but there are certain risk factors that lead to its development. Diabetes is found much more often among four groups of people:[8]

People whose relatives have diabetes. Heredity plays a strong role in the development of diabetes. If you have close relatives who have diabetes, you are five times more likely to develop it than a person who has no diabetic relatives.

People over forty. Diabetes rarely develops in a child under one year of age; it is fairly common among children, and more common among young adults of college age. The most at risk, however, are those over the age of forty.

Women. Two out of every three diabetics are women. For the first twenty-five years of life, there appears to be no substantial difference: Women seem to have diabetes only as often as do men. As age increases, though, so does the difference, until the diabetic rate for women is twice what it is for men among those aged fifty-five to sixty-four. After the age of sixty-four, the difference is again not as great.

Oddly, the higher rate of diabetes among women seems to apply only to women who are or have been married. No one knows the exact reason why, but theories have included causes attributable to the glandular changes during pregnancy (that alter the way the body utilizes starches and sugars), the increase of weight during pregnancy (that many women do not lose after pregnancy), the tendency of previous pregnancies and menopause to put a strain on the glandular system, and the tendency of married women (and men) to eat more than their systems require.

Overweight people. More than 80 percent of those with maturity-onset diabetes were overweight before they developed diabetes. Most are at least 5 percent too heavy when the diabetes is diagnosed, even though the condition causes victims to lose weight. One insurance company found through extensive studies that those who are overweight had one and a half times the death rate from all causes as those of normal weight, and the excess was highest in the case of diabetes: Those who were overweight died from diabetes at four times the normal rate.

Since the earlier diabetes is diagnosed, the better, you should have frequent physical examinations if you fall into one or more of these risk groups; your examinations should always include a test for diabetes.

SYMPTOMS

Many cases of diabetes carry with them no symptoms at all; as mentioned earlier, half of the adults in the United States who have diabetes aren't aware of it. In some cases there may be only mild symptoms, and sometimes there may be only one indication of diabetes. For instance, a victim may simply get tired more easily or may just not feel well. Due to good physical examinations, many cases of diabetes are currently being diagnosed before any symptoms at all appear.

The typical list of symptoms of diabetes includes: excessive thirst, excessive urination, hunger, loss of weight, fatigue (tiring more rapidly and easier than usual), slow healing of cuts and bruises, changes in vision, intense itching, pain in the fingers and toes, or drowsiness. Though these symptoms are the most usual, all of them will not appear in most cases; in many cases the victim may experience only one or two.

Remember, too, that you can have diabetes without having any symptoms at all—a good reason for thorough medical examinations if you are in a high-risk group for developing diabetes.

Diabetes is detected by blood and urine tests; one of the most positive signs of diabetes is high levels of sugar in the blood and urine (since the body is not utilizing glucose and since it remains in the bloodstream until it is eliminated in the urine). Other tests, in cases where the doctor is unsure, measure glucose tolerance by giving the individual a syrupy drink high in sugar content and then testing the urine and blood several times at hourly intervals.

TREATMENT

Most treatment regimes consist of dietary control, injection or ingestion of insulin, and exercise. In about one in three diabetics diet alone is enough to keep the diabetes under control, most often in those who are over the age of forty. When diabetes sets in earlier than the age of forty, it is more likely to be severe and to need more rigorous treatment.

Insulin, generally given by injection under the skin of the arm, abdomen, or thigh, helps lower the amount of sugar in the blood and helps the diabetic utilize some of the blood sugar more efficiently. It is critical that insulin be administered at the proper time of day and that it be administered in the proper dosage; mistakes in administration can lead to diabetic coma (too little insulin) or insulin shock (too much insulin). Either condition, unchecked, can lead to death.

Diabetics are in good control if they feel well, are able to maintain normal weight on a well-balanced diet, have urine tests that are negative (do not indicate high sugar content), and have normal blood tests.

If diabetes is discovered early and if obese victims bring their weight to normal, therapy is sometimes so effective that insulin is no longer needed to control the diabetes.

COPING WITH DIABETES

If you develop diabetes, the suggestions that follow can help make the disease more tolerable.

Follow the diet plan set forth by your doctor. Diet is one of the most important areas of control for diabetes, and diabetics learn to break food groups down into seven exchanges. If you are eating out at a restaurant, you can still follow your dietary restrictions by using some of these tips:[9]

Order vegetable juices, unsweetened fruit juices, clear broth, dill pickles, fresh fruit cocktails, and fresh vegetables for appetizers instead of fish or meat cocktails or canned fruit cocktails. You should order fresh vegetable or fruit salads without the dressings already added, and use a lemon wedge, vinegar, or separate salad dressings.

Vegetables should be ordered stewed, boiled, or steamed; avoid creamed, au gratin, fried, sautéed, or escalloped vegetables. Order your potatoes boiled, steamed, baked, or mashed; stay away from potatoes that are creamed, escalloped, browned, fried, or french fried. Meat, fish, or chicken should be roasted, broiled, boiled, or baked; you should ask that extra fat be trimmed off. Avoid gravy.

Any kind of bread sliced in the average thickness, muffins, biscuits, crackers, corn bread, and hard or soft rolls are fine; stay away from sweet or frosted breads, Danish pastries, coffee cake, and sweet rolls. Desserts should consist of fresh fruit, sponge or angel food cake, or plain ice cream. Custards, candy, frosted cake, pie, or sweetened fruits should not be ordered.

Sweet milk, buttermilk, unsweetened fruit juices, coffee, and tea are acceptable as beverages; don't order soft drinks (exception: low-calorie), milk shakes, chocolate milk, or cocoa.

Overall, cut down on your intake of saturated fats. Trim all the excess fat off meat, avoid fatty cuts of meat (such as pork, lamb, and beef), and use safflower oil or corn oil in place of shortening.

Exercise helps the body utilize sugar and decreases your need for insulin, so develop a program of regular, daily exercise with your doctor's approval. Make sure that your exercise, whatever it is, is regular: Inactivity during the week and a burst of exercise on the weekend can cause your blood sugar to fall to dangerously low levels.

Because diabetes affects the skin and the ability to heal, keep your skin clean and dry. Wash daily with soap and lukewarm water, and pay close attention to your hands, feet, face, and the areas between your legs and under your arms. In areas where the skin creases and bacteria can collect, wash well but gently. Avoid sunburn; use a preparation that keeps out the sun's rays (as listed on the label containing PABA).

If you get a cut, wash the area with soap and water and cover the wound with a sterile bandage. You should check often for signs of infection: throbbing, redness, swelling, or pus. Call your doctor immediately if you detect signs of infection or if the cut does not heal. Do what you can to avoid getting cut; wear gloves if you work around equipment that may cut your hands.

You should have a dental checkup at least once a year; advise your dentist about your diabetes before he or she begins the examination. Brush your teeth after eating and floss daily.

Disorders involving the feet are common with diabetes due to infections, impaired circulation, and progressive loss of sensation in the feet. Keep your feet clean and dry and warm; you should wash them daily with soap and lukewarm water, and you should make sure that they are completely dry—especially between the toes. Change your socks frequently, and if you perspire, dust your feet and socks with cornstarch or talcum powder. Keep your toenails cut short, and cut them straight across to prevent the edges from digging into the skin of your toes. Wear shoes that are comfortable, snug at the heel, wide at the toes, and well made. If you have toes that overlap, use a small piece of lamb's wool to cushion them. Walking and exercising can help improve the circulation to your feet; to help more, avoid sitting with your legs crossed, sitting or standing for too long at a time, and wearing garments or shoes that are too tight.

Check your feet often for blisters, calluses, corns, cuts, burns, or bruises; since you may not have much sensation there, you may hurt yourself without realizing it. Take extra precautions to keep from hurting your feet, and care for any injury you do receive.

If you need to use insulin, buy the preparation and concentration ordered by your doctor. Watch for the expiration date, and don't use the insulin beyond it. You should keep your insulin out of the light, away from freezing temperatures, and away from heat over 95°F. Insulin will keep for weeks at room temperature, but keeping insulin in the refrigerator will slow the growth rate of bacteria; if you keep insulin in the refrigerator, you should remove it at least one hour before you inject it in order to avoid pain and complications. If your insulin is discolored or has particles in it, do not use it. Be sure to keep extra insulin on hand for use in emergencies.

You can inject insulin anywhere on the body where major arteries and nerves are not close to the skin surface and where there is a layer of fatty

115

tissue—especially the upper arms, waistline, thighs, and buttocks. You should make a chart of where you are injecting insulin, and you should not return to the same site for a period of six to eight weeks. You should never make an injection closer than one-half inch from an injection that was made recently.

Many diabetics choose to use disposable syringes; if glass syringes are used, they must be sterilized before each use. To do so, place the forceps, needle, plunger, and barrel in a strainer separately; slowly lower the strainer into a pot of distilled water, and bring the water to boiling. Boil the equipment for ten minutes. After boiling, remove the strainer, pour the water out of the pan, and replace the strainer in the pan and allow the equipment to cool. Once cool, use the forceps to reassemble the syringe; never touch the tips of the forceps, the shaft of the needle, or the sides of the plunger with your fingers. You should hold the needle by the hub, the barrel by the sides, and the plunger by the knob at the top.

Be sure to push out any water that remains in the syringe before you prepare for injection. After injection, force cold water through the assembled syringe to clean the needle; then disassemble the syringe and rinse all the parts with cool tap water.

If you are planning to travel, you will want to make special plans. Carry extra syringes, needles, and insulin; most states require a prescription to purchase insulin, so you should obtain a letter and a prescription from your physician to use in case of emergency. Carry your insulin in an insulated bag, in a briefcase, or on your person; keep it out of car glove compartments and trunks and baggage compartments on trains, buses, and planes.

Keep an emergency supply of sugar on hand; you might consider carrying cookies, orange juice, or candy with you if you go sightseeing, since the exercise accompanying sightseeing can lower your blood sugar.

Check your urine frequently while you travel, and contact your physician or the local chapter of the American Diabetes Association if a problem develops.

ALLERGIES

Even though allergies cause few deaths, they have the capacity for making life miserable.* Experts have conservatively estimated that approximately 35 million Americans—fifteen out of every hundred—suffer from one or more significant allergies. This estimated figure includes those who suffer from hay fever, asthma, and certain other allergies, such as allergic eczema, angioedema (a

*This section adapted in part from *Allergy Research: An Introduction* (Washington, D.C.: U.S. Department of Health, Education and Welfare, Public Health Service, National Institutes of Health), DHEW publication no. (NIH) 72-281.

swelling of body tissue), hives, food allergy, drug allergy, and bee sting allergy. Individuals with contact dermatitis—produced by such agents as poison ivy, poison oak, or poison sumac—and those who in recent years have reported allergic reactions to detergents containing enzyme additives are not included in this figure.

Of all allergic conditions, asthma is usually considered to be the most serious. According to a survey by a private research group, over 38 million patient visits are made each year to private physicians for allergic conditions, and almost one-third of these are for asthma. One-third of all asthma visits are made by children and young adults three to twenty years of age.

According to statistics released by The National Institute of Allergy and Infectious Diseases, an estimated 14.6 million Americans are victims of hay fever, and another 9 million have asthma.[10]

WHAT IS ALLERGY?

Individuals who have an allergy have developed an unusual sensitivity to some substance, known as an allergen, which does not bother most people.* The severity of symptoms resulting from this sensitivity ranges from mildly discomforting to, in rare cases, life-threatening. Common substances that may serve as allergens include foods, drugs, cosmetics, insects, molds, dusts, and pollens. Some of the most common include bees, ragweed, penicillin, chocolate, saccharin, pets, milk, fruits, and nuts.[11]

The allergic process is similar to the immune process, which provides resistance to disease. During an illness caused by an infectious microorganism, specific blood proteins called antibodies form that help protect an individual during future contact with that organism. In the case of allergy, sensitizing antibodies, also known as immunoglobulin E (IgE), are formed during first encounters with an allergen. Upon further exposure to the allergen, IgE antibodies react with certain body cells to bring on the symptoms of an allergic reaction.

Scientists do not yet know what causes one person to develop an allergy to a substance that has no effect on other people. Factors such as a person's ethnic background or sex seem to play no role in the development of allergies. There is evidence, however, that an individual may inherit a tendency to become sensitized but not to any specific allergen.

The most common allergies include hay fever (allergic rhinitis), bronchial asthma, eczema, hives, contact dermatitis, and drug reactions, in order of prevalence.[12]

Pollen Allergy (Bethesda, Md.: Department of Health, Education and Welfare, Public Health Service, National Institutes of Health, National Institute of Allergy and Infectious Diseases, 1976), DHEW publication no. (NIH) 75-493.

HAY FEVER (ALLERGIC RHINITIS)

Allergic rhinitis, the technical name for what is commonly called hay fever, is the most common allergic reaction. Some sufferers have a seasonal form of the disease that causes them to react to specific pollens and mold spores released as trees and shrubbery and other plants bloom and flower. Others have hay fever nearly all year around, reacting to dust, animal dandruff or feathers, musty old books, and musty furniture. Ragweed pollen is the most common offender, followed by other wind-pollenated weeds, grasses, and trees.

The symptoms of hay fever include a stuffy nose with watery (not mucous) discharge; red, itchy eyes; sneezing; a burning, itchy throat; and occasional hearing impairment. There is never fever with hay fever. To tell the difference between a cold and hay fever, check for fever.

There are other ways, too:[13] A cold generally clears up within a week, two at the longest; hay fever lasts and lasts and will return (sometimes in a milder form) the same time each year. A cold can hit anyone of any age; hay fever usually doesn't begin in a person who has reached middle age. There are not itchy eyes with a cold, and your nose doesn't itch with a cold; with hay fever they do. The discharge from the nose is thick and muciferous with a cold; with hay fever it is thin and watery.

If your hay fever is mild, it can generally be treated with such over-the-counter remedies as antihistamines or decongestants. You should always see a doctor if the hay fever is severe or if you experience pain or popping sounds in the ears; persistent coughing; difficulty in breathing; wheezing; or pain above the teeth, in the cheeks, above the eyes, or on the side of the nose. They generally signal complications or something more serious, such as asthma or sinus infection.

BRONCHIAL ASTHMA

Asthma is usually caused by some kind of allergy, and it is the most serious of the allergic reactions; each year several thousand victims die from asthma and its complications.[14] About 9 million Americans—about 4 percent of the population—suffer from asthma and the majority of them are children.[15]

Asthma victims are generally extremely sensitive to such allergens as dust, pollens, fungi, animal dandruff, cold air, air pollutants, and even certain foods. Asthmatic attacks that are related specifically to seasonal allergies are usually seasonal in nature, just as hay fever is; it is common for victims to have both hay fever and asthma. Not all asthmatics have asthma because of allergy; about 20 percent have asthma caused by other factors.

The symptoms of asthma include coughing, wheezing, and extremely labored breathing. Because the victim cannot get enough air to oxygenate the blood properly, he or she develops a bluish tint of the skin, lips, and fingernails (called cyanosis). In severe cases, the chest appears to be overly expanded, and the victim gasps for air.

118

Most asthma begins in childhood; and about 30 percent of all children who have asthma also have eczema (another allergic reaction). An infant who has both asthma and eczema has a greatly increased chance of having asthma as a permanent condition than an infant whose asthma is not accompanied by eczema. Approximately half of the children who have asthma when they enter kindergarten do not have it as adults; the attacks become less and less frequent and severe as time goes by. Only about 5 to 10 percent of childhood asthmatics still have severe asthma as adults.

Even those who develop asthma as adults do not necessarily have it for the rest of their lives.

Possibly because the nervous system increases sensitivity, asthma attacks are more frequent and more severe during times of emotional stress or intense nervousness.

Most asthma can be controlled by medication and exercise.

ECZEMA

Characterized by skin eruptions, itching, swelling, blistering, oozing, and scaling, eczema often begins in the bends of the elbows and knees (especially in babies) and occasionally spreads to involve the entire body.

The chief cause of eczema in infants is a reaction to food, especially cow's milk and eggs. Adults commonly react to soaps, pollens, and a number of foods.

Women are more prone to eczema because their skin is more sensitive than men's skin; fair skin is more susceptible than is dark skin.[16] Sensitivity of the skin is also influenced by the general state of health, emotional stress, and excessive perspiration.

HIVES

Hives, sometimes called urticaria, are itchy swollen areas that look like welts. They can be as small as a pinhead or as large as a coin; they can be confined to a small area, or they can spread over the entire body. In severe cases giant hives may cause extreme swelling of the mouth, tongue, feet, or other parts of the body.

Most of the time hives are caused by allergy, usually to food or drugs. In some cases, however, hives are the result of infection or emotional stress.

CONTACT DERMATITIS

Occurring most commonly on the hands, legs, face, and neck, contact dermatitis is an allergic reaction of the skin caused by allergens that come in contact with the skin—usually deodorants, detergents, cosmetics, and dyes. The skin becomes inflamed and itchy; poison ivy and poison oak cause contact dermatitis. (Contrary to belief, not everyone who contacts poison ivy will get a rash; the person must have more than one contact with the weed and must build up a sensitivity to it.)

Contact dermatitis may go away in a few minutes, or it may last several hours or several days. It may appear as a patch of redness or a fine rash, or it may involve inflammation that extends to the eyelids, tongue, hands, and feet. In extreme cases the entire body may swell. In some cases tiny blood vessels under the skin surface may leak, producing purplish-red bruiselike marks called purpura.

Most cases of contact dermatitis are localized; the rash, bumps, swelling, and blisters develop on the skin that actually came in contact with the allergen.

FOOD AND DRUGS

When foods that act as allergens come in contact with the lining of the digestive tract, they can cause local reactions such as sores in the mouth, spasms of the stomach or intestines (such as colic, which occurs frequently in infants), or diarrhea. When the allergens enter the bloodstream as a natural part of digestion, reactions can occur anywhere in the body.

Milk is the most common offender. Next, in order of prevalence, come eggs, fish, shellfish, wheat, berries, nuts, pork, chocolate, beans, peanuts, and fresh fruits (such as tomatoes and strawberries). If you are sensitive to one fruit or vegetable or food, you will likely be sensitive to others of the same family. For instance, if you react to brussels sprouts, you will also probably react to mustard, radishes, broccoli, and cabbage. Many are allergic to one or more of the more than three thousand additives, colorings, and preservatives used in processing food.

The most usual symptoms of food allergy include constipation, diarrhea, cramps, indigestion, vomiting, and/or nausea. The effects may begin a few minutes after you eat the food, or it may take hours or days for the reaction to occur.

Reactions to drugs can range from mild to severe and can even include a fatal condition called anaphylactic shock. The reactions may occur within minutes or, like food allergies, may take hours or days to occur. Symptoms include rash, hives, general itching, widespread red and scaly eruptions, and oval or round welts that always appear at the site where the drug was injected. In severe cases, the victim may experience difficulty in breathing and tightening of the throat and chest.

Penicillins and other drugs of the sulfa group are the most common offenders.

INSECT BITES AND STINGS

Each year in the United States, insect stings kill about fifty people, and thousands of other victims react with such violence that they require hospitalization or other medical care.[17]* Some think that the death estimate is too conserva-

*This section for the most part adapted from Alvin Silverstein and Virginia B. Silverstein, *Allergies* (Philadelphia: J. B. Lippincott Company, 1977), pp. 78–85.

tive, citing evidence that some deaths attributed to cardiac arrest or convulsions may actually be due to insect stings. Most who do die from insect stings die within twenty minutes of the sting.

Most common among the culprits include honeybees, hornets, wasps, yellow jackets, and ants. Less serious reactions occur to bites or stings of mosquitos, bloodsucking flies, fleas, and other biting insects.

You should suspect an allergic reaction if you experience any of the following symptoms following a sting or bite: swelling of unusual size or duration at the sting site, hives, overall itching, tightness in the chest, abdominal pain, nausea or vomiting, dizziness, weakness, speech difficulties, and a feeling of uneasiness or malaise. In extreme cases of anaphylactic shock the blood pressure will drop rapidly and unconsciousness results. If you experience any of these symptoms, you should get to a doctor or hospital *immediately*.

There are some things you can do to lessen the pain involved in an insect sting that causes only a mild reaction. Wash the area around the sting site promptly with soap and water; remove the stinger, and don't squeeze it, since you will pump more venom into your skin. The best method of stinger removal is to scrape it away from the skin with a knife or your fingernail; remove it as soon as possible, because it will continue pumping venom even after it has torn away from the insect's body. Apply ice or cold packs to the sting site to help keep the venom from spreading; meat tenderizer, promptly applied to the sting, can help break down the venom. Elevate the area of the sting to help decrease circulation, and avoid exercise and rapid movement. You may want to take antihistamines to sooth itching, and pain-killing ointments applied directly to the skin may ease the pain of the sting.

DIGESTIVE DISEASES

More Americans are hospitalized because of diseases of the stomach, liver, intestines, pancreas, and other parts of the gastrointestinal tract than because of any other group of disorders.[18] Digestive diseases affect nearly 18 million Americans, ranking second only to cardiovascular diseases in number of physician office visits or house calls and responsible for 245 million days per year of restricted activity. The total cost of illness resulting from digestive diseases is approaching $11.5 billion a year.

HEARTBURN

Heartburn—which has nothing to do with the heart—is one of the most common complaints of gastrointestinal origin. The lower esophageal sphincter (LES), a band of muscle at the end of the esophagus where it joins the stomach, functions to open and let food pass into the stomach; normally, the LES closes when food is not passing through to prevent stomach contents from being regurgitated back into the esophagus.

In some individuals—no one knows why—the LES is weak, and it opens and relaxes, allowing regurgitation of the stomach's hydrochloric acid into the esophagus, where it irritates the sensitive mucous lining of the esophagus.

Current research is centering on the development of new drugs, chemical methods, and surgical methods of correcting weak or malfunctioning LES.

HIATAL HERNIA

Another condition resulting from a weak LES, hiatal hernia causes a weakness of the esophagus where it joins the stomach; as a result, part of the stomach protrudes into the chest cavity.

PEPTIC ULCER

Peptic ulcer, one of the nation's most serious health problems, afflicts about 15 million—or nearly 7 percent of the population—in this country alone.* Every day about 4,000 more individuals develop an ulcer, and each year some 12,000 die in the United States of complications of peptic ulcer. It has been estimated that lost workhours and medical expenses due to peptic ulcer cause a $1-billion annual drain on the economy.

A peptic ulcer is a noncancerous, craterlike sore called an erosion in the wall of the stomach or intestine; the ulcer erodes through the thin, inner mucous membrane lining of the stomach or intestine and into the deeper muscular wall. Peptic ulcers occur only in those regions of the gastrointestinal tract that are bathed by the digestive juices secreted by the stomach, and derive their name from the protein-digesting enzyme, pepsin.

Almost all peptic ulcers occur either in the stomach itself or in the small intestine just below the stomach. Those located in the first portion of the small intestine are called duodenal ulcers, and those in the stomach are called gastric ulcers. In the United States duodenal ulcers are about eight times more common than gastric ulcers.

The hydrochloric acid and pepsin secreted by the stomach bring about the digestion of meat and other proteins as they reach the stomach. Under normal conditions the mucous membrane lining of the stomach and duodenum is resistant to the digestive mixture, and no ulcer develops. In some people, however, this resistance breaks down and an ulcer forms. The controlling factors, then, are the amount of acid and pepsin secreted by the stomach and the ability of the intestinal wall to resist erosion from the mixture.

Of these two factors, the secretion of too much acid and pepsin is by far the

*This section adapted from U.S. Department of Health, Education and Welfare, *Peptic Ulcer* (Washington, D.C.: U.S. Government Printing Office, 1977), DHEW publication no. (NIH) 72-38, pp. 4–7.

most important. The great majority of people with duodenal ulcers and some of the people with gastric ulcers secrete much more acid than does the normal person. Excretion of excess acid is the most readily controllable by medical techniques.

The large middle portion of the stomach—called the body of the stomach—is lined with cells that produce acid and pepsin. Two important triggers stimulate these cells to secrete more acid: stimulation by the vagus nerve (as a response to hunger, the sight or smell of food, or tension and anxiety) and the presence of food in the lower part of the stomach or duodenum. As a result, a person who is tense most of the time will secrete more acid—not only when his or her stomach has food in it but when it's empty as well, due to stimulation by the vagus nerve responding to anxiety.

Specific foods and many drugs can greatly increase the amount of acid and may also be directly irritating to the stomach and duodenal walls. Alcohol, coffee, and aspirin are notorious examples of this type of irritant.

Symptoms of ulcer can vary, but the most common, almost universal symptom of peptic ulcer is pain—usually steady, and often resembling a burning or gnawing in the stomach. The pain often feels like it is in a small area of the abdomen, usually somewhere between the navel and the lower end of the breastbone. The pain generally appears from thirty minutes to two hours after a meal, and it is usually relieved if you eat more food or take an antacid. Some ulcer sufferers have pain of this kind that occurs off and on for years.

Risks. Almost anyone is at risk for developing a peptic ulcer; they can occur any time from infancy to old age and are most frequent in people who are twenty years old or older. People in their thirties, forties, and fifties are slightly more prone to develop gastric ulcer than are people who are sixty or older, but when they do develop in older people, they are generally more serious. Ulcers in this country occur more frequently in men than in women, although peptic ulcer is increasing in frequency among women.

You have particular risk of developing ulcer if you are under continuous strain of any kind, regardless of your age or sex.

If members of your immediate family have gastric or duodenal ulcers, you are slightly more prone to develop one yourself, but your tendency is probably simply due to the anxiety-ridden environment in the family. It is very possible that if you have close blood relatives with ulcers, you will never develop one yourself.

Complications. There are three major complications of gastric and duodenal ulcers: narrowing and obstruction, hemorrhage, and perforation.

Ulcers that lie in the duodenum or in the narrow section of the stomach where it meets the duodenum may become inflamed and swollen or become surrounded by scar tissue, causing the intestinal opening to become narrow or closed. Such an intestinal obstruction keeps food from passing from the stomach, and the victim vomits his or her meals or constantly regurgitates the secretions of the stomach. In most cases surgery is necessary to correct the condition.

As an ulcer erodes into the muscular portion of the intestinal wall, it damages blood vessels there and may cause bleeding. If the damaged blood vessels are small, the blood will ooze out slowly and over a long period of time, and the victim will become anemic. On the other hand, if the damaged blood vessel is large, the hemorrhage that results is rapid and very dangerous. The patient may feel light-headed and faint or may collapse suddenly. Prompt medical attention is critical and should consist of transfusion and possible surgery; if medical attention is not obtained, the victim could bleed to death internally. If you notice tarry black blood in the stools, you should report to your doctor immediately.

Occasionally an ulcer will erode all the way through the wall of the stomach or duodenum, and partially digested food from the digestive tract and bacteria that is normally present in the digestive tract spill out into the sterile abdominal cavity, resulting in peritonitis. A sudden perforation causes severe pain throughout most of the abdomen. Perforations, like hemorrhage, are medical emergencies and require prompt medical attention, usually including surgery.

Treatment for uncomplicated peptic ulcer is generally aimed at decreasing the amount of acid or irritants that reach the stomach and interfere with the normal healing process.

There is usually some restriction in diet, and the amount and degree depend on the individual and the ulcer. A small ulcer that causes only moderate discomfort may heal if the victim eliminates alcohol, coffee, and other irritating foods; cuts down on smoking; and eats a few crackers or drinks a little milk when he feels pain. Ulcers that have progressed and that cause a severe amount of pain, however, may prompt a physician to order small meals on an hourly schedule. Those with severe ulcers are generally ordered to maintain a bland diet.

Any person with an active ulcer should avoid alcohol, coffee, heavily spiced food, excessive smoking, and irritating drugs such as aspirin.

There are over five hundred types of antacids on the market, and you can generally find one that is pleasant to take and that your doctor will approve. Antacids work by neutralizing the hydrochloric acid in the stomach.

Your physician may also prescribe belladonna or a similar drug that blocks the passage of acid-stimulating impulses down the vagus nerve to the stomach.

One of the most important—and difficult—parts of therapy is successfully reducing tension and worry. You should, among other things, avoid taking on more responsibilities than time allows for, take time out for leisure, get a sufficient amount of rest, and avoid situations you know are stressful.

If you are unsuccessful in reducing the amount of stress you suffer, your physician may prescribe a tranquilizer, a mild sedative, or even a term of hospital rest.

In severe instances, when the ulcer will not heal or when there has been hemorrhage or perforation, surgery is usually required.

APPENDICITIS

A narrow tubular attachment to the colon, the appendix is considered to be a vestigial organ—an organ that has degenerated through disuse. The guinea pig, the rabbit, and the rat, among others, have a fully functioning appendix that is used to digest hard seeds, bulk foods, and grasses. In humans, however, the appendix appears to have no function in the digestive process.

In some cases the appendix becomes irritated and inflamed; in certain instances the inflammation results from obstruction due to partially undigested food blocking the appendix, but in many instances the cause of inflammation is unknown. As the inflammation increases, pressure builds up, and the appendix becomes even more inflamed.

Increasing pressure and inflammation can eventually cause the appendix to rupture, spilling bacteria and other foreign matter into the sterile abdominal cavity, resulting in peritonitis; the peritonitis can be fatal if the patient does not receive prompt medical attention. Emergency surgery is necessary to drain the infection and remove the diseased organ from the body.

If appendicitis is diagnosed before the appendix ruptures, as happens in most cases, the diseased appendix is removed through a small incision in the abdominal wall. Appendectomies are no longer considered to be major surgery, and most patients recover without any complications. If the appendix ruptures and peritonitis results, the prognosis is worse: Of the 1,100 who die yearly of appendicitis, almost 1,000 have peritonitis.

Symptoms. In most cases the victim has an attack of acute pain that starts in the center of the abdomen. As the appendicitis worsens, the pain gradually intensifies and moves to the lower right side of the abdomen. Nausea, vomiting, and fever are usually present.

Though some flareups of appendicitis may subside and symptoms may disappear, the only permanent treatment for the condition is surgical removal of the diseased organ.

INFECTIOUS DISEASES

Infectious diseases—or contagious, or communicable, diseases, as they are sometimes called—have been with us through history and will probably always be with us. Common usage has made all of the foregoing terms interchangeable, but, strictly speaking, *infectious* diseases include any disease that is caused by a living organism, regardless of the way the disease is transmitted. A contagious, or communicable, disease, on the other hand, is one that is spread by *direct contact* with the infectious agents that cause the disease.[19]

THE NATURE
OF INFECTIOUS DISEASES

An infection—a state when an organism capable of causing disease is present and multiplying within the body—is produced when body tissues are invaded by microorganisms that multiply and result in the signs and symptoms of disease. In many cases a local infection may be present at the same time a generalized infection—one that spreads in the bloodstream throughout the entire body—is present.[20]

OCCURRENCE OF DISEASE

There are various kinds and occurrences involving disease, and medical researchers have coined several terms to describe the prevalence of any certain disease.[21]

Sporadic is the term used to describe a disease that occurs at varying intervals—not permanently. A sporadic disease affects only a few people.

An *endemic* disease is constantly present in a given community, but it affects only a few people at any given time.

An *epidemic* is an unusual and sudden occurrence of a disease that affects many people, but only for a limited amount of time. A *pandemic* is a disease of epidemic proportions—affecting many people for a limited amount of time—that involves several countries of the world, or, in severe cases, all countries of the world.

THE INFECTIOUS PROCESS

In order for infection to occur and disease to be spread, a chain of events needs to be completed—including the presence of an infectious agent, a source of the infectious agent (called a *reservoir*), a way for the infectious agent to escape from the reservoir, a way for the infectious agent to travel to the new host (mode of transmission), a way for the infectious agent to enter the new host (mode of entry), and a susceptible new host.

INFECTIOUS AGENTS

The first link of the chain—the presence of an infectious agent—includes several major groups of microorganisms that are responsible for infection and resultant disease in man. The infectious agent lives and multiplies at the expense of the host and to the host's detriment.

There are seven major groups of microorganisms that act as infectious agents.

Parasites. Parasites, which invade the body and cause infection, are visible only under a microscope. In some conditions—referred to as infestation—the parasites involved are large enough to be seen with the naked eye.

Viruses. Viruses invade living cells and multiply within those cells; an ultramicroscopic form of life, they cause diseases that have characteristics distinguishing them from diseases caused by other agents. Influenza, rabies, measles, smallpox, and mumps are common conditions caused by viruses.

Bacteria. Bacteria are single-celled organisms; unlike viruses, which multiply within body cells, bacteria multiply by simple cellular division and are capable of growing outside living tissue. Even when in tissue, bacteria do not invade the cells but grow instead on the surfaces of cells or between cells. The mode of attack is from outside the cell, not from the inside. Bacterial infections are responsive to treatment with antibiotics; viral infections are not.

Rickettsiae. Rickettsiae, smaller than true bacteria, live within the body cells of the host and they require living cells in order to multiply and grow. Rickettsiae cause such diseases as Rocky Mountain spotted fever and typhus.

Fungi and molds. Not all fungi cause disease, but some are critical elements in certain kinds of diseases—such as a number of infections of the skin (including ringworm and athlete's foot).

Protozoa. Protozoa are one-celled animal forms such as the amoebae, the trypanosomes, and the plasmodia. One disease caused by protozoan invasion is amoebic dysentery, an acute form of diarrhea.

Metazoa. Metazoa are animals of more than one cell; some that commonly cause disease include hookworms, tapeworms, and pinworms. Trichinella, often present in raw pork, can cause trichinosis if the pork that is eaten is not cooked thoroughly.

Symptoms and signs of disease result when an organism either directly invades the cells or causes toxins that in turn invade and poison the cells and body systems.

SOURCE OF INFECTIOUS AGENT (RESERVOIR OF INFECTION)

Sources—or reservoirs—of infection can be human, animal, or environmental.

Most of the infectious diseases that are harmful to man originate from human sources; a human source may be simply a carrier—able to infect others without experiencing symptoms or signs himself—or may manifest signs or symptoms that range in severity all the way to a frank manifestation of the disease. In some instances there are missed cases—examples where both the patient and the doctor fail to diagnose the patient as having the disease at all. In other cases the disease may be atypical: The disease may not manifest the usual signs and symptoms but is still diagnosed. In still other cases the patient may recover before all the signs or symptoms occur (a condition referred to as abortive disease).

People who are carriers of disease may harbor the infection and spread it to others before their own signs and symptoms occur (incubationary carriers, infectious during the incubation period), or may harbor the infection and spread it to others after they themselves have recovered from the disease (convalescent carriers).

Carriers are just as important a factor in the spread of disease as are those who are literally ill with the disease. In some cases of illness—meningitis, for example—the number of carriers far exceeds the number who are ill with the disease, so many are unknowingly exposed. Other diseases, such as measles, are not communicable unless the carrier has developed symptoms.

Animals that can serve as sources of infection for man include fish, birds, lobsters, shrimp, crabs, water fleas, fleas, flies, lice, bees, spiders, mites, ticks, slugs, snails, oysters, clams, mussels, and such mammals as rats, cattle, horses, bats, swine, cats, dogs, and monkeys.

Some infectious agents live in the soil, and the environment is the main source of infection. The fungi that cause a number of diseases and the molds that are found in soil and dust or on vegetation in areas where disease is common can serve as sources of infection for a number of disorders.

ESCAPE OF ORGANISMS FROM RESERVOIR

The mere existence of an infectious agent does not guarantee that disease will result, because the infectious agent must first find an avenue of escape and leave its old host before it can attack a new one.[22]

The most common—and the most dangerous—avenue of escape is through the respiratory tract, facilitated by coughing, sneezing, speaking, and even exhaling tiny droplets that contain infectious organisms. Droplets can be driven many feet if expelled in a cough or sneeze; they can be carried even farther by the wind. Even the act of normal conversation carries droplets several feet.[23]

A second common avenue of escape is through the intestinal tract—chiefly through the feces but sometimes through the urine. Urine carries far fewer disease agents than do feces. Organisms may escape through draining lesions, through discharges from the urethra, or through vaginal discharge.

Still another mode of escape involves an external force, such as an insect, who bites or sucks infected blood and then transmits the disease to others.

Some agents never leave their hosts; for example, the larvae of the pork worm that causes trichinosis never leaves the live pork but escapes only if a new host eats the infected pork tissue. In other diseases the infectious agent cannot leave its host at certain stages in its development; for example, there is no spread of the bacteria that cause syphilis when the host is in the late stages.

There is usually only a single avenue of escape, but there may be more in some instances—such as smallpox, in which the infectious agents escape from the host through both skin lesions and the respiratory tract.

MODES OF TRANSMISSION

The spread of disease depends on the ability of the infectious agent to survive outside its source. Transmission of the agent may be direct or indirect and is dependent on favorable factors to be successful.

Direct transmission methods include droplet spread, in which the infected person sprays the face of a noninfected person by sneezing, coughing, or talking; direct contact with the infected person, usually accomplished through kissing or sexual intercourse; and fecal-oral spread, accomplished generally when the hands are contaminated with soiled clothing, bedding, or towels and then are put in contact with the mouth.

Indirect transmission involves vehicles—nonliving means of transmission—and vectors—animate or living means of transmission. The most common include polluted water (responsible for cholera, amoebic dysentery, and typhoid fever), milk (usually spread from infected cattle, responsible for typhoid fever, scarlet fever, and diphtheria), food that has been improperly refrigerated or cooked, air (which carries droplets, dust, and aerosols responsible for the common cold, influenza, whooping cough, measles, and chicken pox), soil, bedding, clothing, doorknobs, and drinking fountains.

ENTRY OF ORGANISM INTO NEW HOST

The portal of entry into the new host is often the same as the portal of exit from the old host. The most common portals of entry exist in four major body systems:

The respiratory system. Organisms enter the body through the mouth, nose, pharynx, larynx, trachea, bronchi, and lungs.

The skin. Unbroken skin is a barrier to infection in most cases; rare exceptions include the ability of hookworms to burrow through the soles of the feet. Most infection enters the body through broken skin and through mucous membranes, including the conjunctiva.

The gastrointestinal system. The mouth, pharynx, and nose are also points of entry involving the gastrointestinal system. Others include the stomach, the small and large intestines, the rectum, and the anus. Also included are the organs of digestion: the pancreas, liver, gallbladder, and salivary glands.

The genitourinary system. In the woman, agents of infection can enter the body through the ovaries, vagina, uterus, and fallopian tubes; in the man they can enter through the testes, prostate gland, seminal vesicles, spermatic duct, and epididymis. In both sexes infectious agents may enter the body through the kidneys, bladder, urethra, or ureters.

In some cases the point of entry is in the same organ or system that is affected by the disease; in other cases an infectious agent may enter the body through a mode of entry that bears no relationship to the eventual course of the disease.

SUSCEPTIBILITY OF HOST

In order for the cycle of disease to occur, the new host must be susceptible to the disease; for example, a measles virus may be transmitted successfully to a new host, but if the new host has developed an immunity (either through vaccination or through a former experience with measles), there will be no resulting disease.

A human being may be able to resist disease for a number of reasons:

There may be mechanical barriers, such as the skin when it is unbroken. The mucous membranes of the respiratory, gastrointestinal tract, and genitourinary tract may serve as barriers if they are in a healthy condition.

Certain cells of the blood and cells found in the liver, spleen, lymph nodes, and bone marrow engulf and destroy invading infectious agents and remove them from the body in a process called *phagocytosis*.

Many body secretions either trap infecting organisms, wash them away, or destroy them. Perspiration, mucous, the digestive juices found in the stomach or intestines, tears, and urine all act as protective agents; in many instances, the saliva aids to prevent infection.

If the new host has had previous experiences with the infecting agent, he or she will have developed an acquired immunity that will prevent reinfection with the same infectious agent. Immunity can be developed after having the disease or may be developed as a result of vaccination or immunization—introduction of the antigens into the system and subsequent building of immunity.

IMMUNIZATION

There is protection available against some of the most serious infectious diseases. Tragically, too many people aren't taking advantage of that protection: Even though a vaccine is readily available, the incidence of whooping cough in the United States doubled in two recent years. Polio outbreaks continue, and seventeen victims were crippled in the United States in 1977. That same year over

57,000 children came down with measles—not a harmless childhood disease, but an affliction that can lead to brain inflammation, blindness, brain damage, deafness, mental retardation, pneumonia, encephalitis, and death in one out of every thousand children who get it.[24]

There are seven vaccinations or immunizations that everyone should have —diphtheria, pertussis, tetanus, polio, rubella, mumps, and measles. You need others if you are going to travel abroad into areas where disease has been recent.

MEASLES (RUBEOLA)

Called the red measles, rubeola is one of the most serious diseases a child can have: Complications include brain inflammation and death and can leave a child deaf and blind. Once, 90 percent of the red measles cases occurred in children under the age of ten; now young adults account for more than 60 percent of the red measles cases in the United States. The problem? It's the older victims—those in high school and college—who are particularly vulnerable to encephalitis as a complication.[25]

GERMAN MEASLES (RUBELLA)

In children the German measles are often so mild that in many cases they go undetected. In other cases they may be misdiagnosed as a simple cold or some other mild disorder.

But when German measles strike a woman in the first trimester of pregnancy, the disease wrecks havoc on the fetus and can result in cerebral palsy, blindness, congenital heart defects, cataracts, arthritis, encephalitis, deafness, and mental retardation. The woman may have a miscarriage, or the baby may die in the uterus.

Vaccination is recommended for previously unvaccinated adolescents, and for women and girls who are not pregnant at the time. You should avoid pregnancy for three months after you have been vaccinated. It's a good idea to get a vaccination even if you think you may have had the disease as a child.

Rubeola vaccine should be administered at fifteen months; a booster is needed in certain cases during adolescence. The German measles vaccine should be administered from twelve to fifteen months (given at fifteen months if combined with measles and mumps vaccinations). Adolescents and adults who are not pregnant and who do not have high fever can be vaccinated at any time.

POLIO

Currently millions of children under the age of fourteen are still unprotected from polio, and outbreaks still occur in the United States and other areas of the world. Adults who are exposed to unusual risk should be immunized, as should adults who are not immunized as children. The most widely used form of polio vaccination is the oral method. The vaccine is given in a series of four doses and should be started when the child is two months old.

MAJOR INFECTIOUS DISEASES

Disease	Pathogen	How Transmitted	Incubation Period	Characteristics of Occurrence
Botulism	Bacteria	Contaminated food not properly canned	Often less than 24 hours	Most outbreaks in U.S. are attributed to home-canned nonacid vegetables. *C. botulinum* is frequently found in garden soil. Its spores are extremely heat-resistant. Organisms in improperly canned foods can generate toxin. Fortunately the *toxin* is destroyed by boiling a few minutes. The majority of cases are caused by Type A or B organisms. There are six strains of botulism.
Chickenpox (varicella)	Virus	Spreads by air, through inhalation; droplets are directly or indirectly spread.	14-16 days	Occurs epidemically, mainly in winter and spring, before age 20; affects both sexes equally. Virus reaches skin from respiratory system via the blood. Virus can affect nerve pathways, causing the disease "shingles" years after the infection.
Cholera	Bacteria	By direct contact with patients in incubation stage; food, utensils, and water contaminated by fecal materials; flies.	1-3 days	Cholera is endemic in certain Asian countries. Few cases occur in the U.S. Travelers to countries where cholera is endemic or epidemic should be immunized before departure.
Diphtheria	Bacteria	Directly by droplet infection from respiratory discharges, and through contamination of hands, objects and, occasionally, milk.	2-5 days	Endemic and epidemic where child immunization measures have been neglected.
Encephalitis Viral (arthopod-borne)	Virus	By mosquitoes that feed on birds harboring the virus (without suffering any ill effects).	5-15 days	Three types of encephalitis viruses cause the bulk of the infections in the U.S.: Eastern equine, St. Louis, and Western. The types of birds that harbor the disease vary, as do the types of mosquitoes, but the latter's bite is the source of the virus for man, as well as for horses, mules, and other mammals.
Hepatitis, Infectious	Virus	Fecal or oral discharges contaminating food, water, or milk.	15-35 days	Occurs sporadically and in small local epidemics which have been traced to sewage-contaminated water or consumption of contaminated food, especially shellfish. It is believed that, like serum hepatitis, infectious hepatitis may also be transmitted by injection equipment.

Signs and Symptoms	Prevention
Vomiting, constipation, double vision, thirst, difficulty in swallowing, paralysis of pharynx, labored breathing, secretion of thick saliva. Temperature normal or subnormal. Death results from respiratory failure.	Proper canning of meats and vegetables; boil all home-canned, nonacid food before serving.
Mild disease with fever and itching vesicular eruption. Papules make appearance about 24 hours after onset of fever. Lesions are most abundant over the trunk, but also on the face, and spread to mouth, throat, and extremities. Successive crops of lesions may be seen, with general involvement of lymph glands.	Immunizations (somewhat ineffective); gamma globulin prevents some cases.
Sudden onset. Copious and frequent watery stools and prostration. Vomiting. Severe dehydration. Loss of as much as 15% of body weight in a few hours. Thirst, but patient cannot retain fluids or food. Features become pinched, eyes sunken. Painful cramps. Enfeebled voice. Rapid and weak pulse, low blood pressure. Uremia. Death may sometimes occur in a few hours.	Cholera vaccine is effective for a few months.
Abrupt fever, chilliness, malaise, sore throat. Whitish-grey membrane forms on tonsils and then thickens to form yellowish diphtheric membrane. Other areas may also be invaded. Cervical lymph nodes are swollen. Bacteria do not invade the tissues but produce toxins that cause heart and kidney damage.	Diphtheria-pertussis-tetanus toxoids (DPT) and diphtheria-tetanus toxoids (D-T) for pediatric use, and special tetanus and diphtheria toxoids (T-D) for adult use.
The severity of encephalitic symptoms varies. In the St. Louis type, high fever, vomiting, headache, vertigo, nuchal ragidity, ataxia, and confusion are among the more serious symptoms. The Western equine type may involve repeated convulsions and deep coma.	
Headache, fever, and anorexia (in most cases), shaking chills (in half). Nausea and vomiting. Malaise, myalgia (sore muscles), joint stiffness, sore throat, dull upper abdominal pain. Urine darkens. Jaundice. Most cases recover fully within four months. Disease tends to be mild in children and young adults; more serious in older adults.	Gamma globulin after known exposure is helpful but does not prevent the disease.

133

Disease	Pathogen	How Transmitted	Incubation Period	Characteristics of Occurrence
Hepatitis, Serum	Virus	Inadequately sterilized needles and syringes; blood or blood products.	2-6 mos.; 12-14 weeks average	The virus may circulate in the blood for eight years or more after the patient has recovered. Tests can now detect the virus in the blood and are a means of preventing spread of disease by transfusion.
Herpes Simplex	Virus	Presumably by direct or droplet contact, and maybe by indirect association.	Unknown	Primary herpes simplex is mainly a disease of childhood. In adults, herpes-like episodes may occur during attacks of pneumonia, meningitis, malaria, and other diseases. The virus lives in balance with most tissues and does not reveal its presence until some stress shifts the balance in favor of the virus.
Herpes Zoster (shingles)	Virus	Perhaps by air or contact from children with chickenpox; sometimes accompanies pneumonia and tuberculosis.	7-14 days	Sporadic occurrence, especially in winter and spring, rarely seen before age 20. Occurs more often in males than in females.
Infectious Mononucleosis	Virus	Direct contact, secretions.	4-14 days	Outbreaks in colleges, camps, and institutions, but generally appears sporadically. Typically affects young adults. Very little is known about the disease.
Influenza	Virus	Droplet infection, soiled articles, direct contact.	24-72 hours	Sporadic cases, local epidemics, pandemics. May affect up to 50% of population within period of 4-6 weeks. Each year the National Institutes of Health, after a careful survey of viruses recovered from recent influenza cases, decides what the exact composition and strength of influenza vaccine should be for the new season, and that becomes the new standard for all U.S. manufacturers.
Measles (Rubeola)	Virus	Respiratory discharges directly or indirectly.	9-11 days	Most outbreaks in late winter and early spring. Epidemics run in 2 to 3 year cycles. Mainly a disease of children; mortality is highest in those under 5 years old and in the aged.
German Measles (Rubella)	Virus	Respiratory discharges directly or indirectly.	9-11 days	Usually a childhood disease, it is fairly common in adults. One attack may confer lifelong immunity. The age group usually affected is from 2 to 15 years. Permanent effects are rare except for damage to the unborn child when the mother is infected in the first 6 months of pregnancy.
Mumps	Virus	Infected droplets or direct contact with salivary droplets from infected person.	17-21 days	Mumps occur most often in the 5-15 age group, but disease may attack adults. Because of the low degree of infectivity, many adults have not been exposed to the disease, and are susceptible. Many cases are asymptomatic.

Symptoms resemble those of infectious hepatitis, but are more severe.

Proper blood storage and sterilization techniques; gamma globulin for all persons over age 40 receiving blood transfusions is recommended by some.

The commonest form of the disease is characterized by painful blisters on lips and gums sometimes associated with fever, irritability, malaise, and swelling of glands. Symptoms may persist for 7 to 10 days. Other sites sometimes affected are the genitalia, and the conjunctivae and eye. It is likely that most herpes simplex-like attacks in adults are caused by other, as yet ill-defined, viruses.

Onset often marked by severe pain, fever, malaise, and tenderness. Affected area develops small blisters that are often moist and weeping.

Malaise, fever, lymphatic enlargement (neck). Some have jaundice due to hepatitis (difficult to distinguish from infectious hepatitis).

Sudden onset, fever of 1-7 days, chills, listlessness, nausea, vomiting, prostration, aches and pains in back and limbs, coryza, sore throat, bronchitis.

Immunization for high risk individuals, i.e., those with diabetes, chronic respiratory diseases, heart ailments, advanced age.

Rhinitis, cough, mild fever, headache, malaise, fatigue, anorexia, conjunctivitis, eye sensitivity to light, and lacrimation. Rash usually appears the second to the fourth day.

Immunization.

Mild rash, slight fever, and swelling of lymph nodes. These symptoms usually appear from 14 to 21 days after exposure and last for only 1 to 4 days.

Immunization; gamma globulin may curtail symptoms; the vaccine should not be given to pregnant women.

Prodromal symptoms (fever, chilliness, malaise, loss of appetite, and headache) may or may not precede swelling of parotid gland. Swelling may affect one or two glands, with tenderness and difficulty in moving jaw. Testes, ovaries, pancreas or thyroid gland can also be involved.

Immunizations are available but do not offer full immunity.

135

Disease	Pathogen	How Transmitted	Incubation Period	Characteristics of Occurrence
Pertussis (whooping cough)	Bacteria	Inhalation of droplets or dusts from infected person.	7-14 days	Epidemic at 2 to 4 year intervals; endemic in winter and spring; mainly disease of infants and very young children; high mortality under six months of age. Highly contagious.
Plague	Bacteria	Fleas (from wild rodents), not directly communicable.	2-10 days	Endemic in Asia, plague sometimes appears in parts of Africa and South America. Ground squirrels and prairie dogs in the western states of the U.S. have been found infected; these animals can transmit plague to "domestic" rats, and thence to man. Disease is spread principally by migration in rat-infested ships.
Poliomyelitis	Virus	Nose and mouth droplets, as well as fecal contamination.	7-14 days	Children most susceptible; pregnant women vulnerable. Mild infections confer full immunity. There are three strains of virus.
Rabies	Virus	Bites of rabid animals, mainly dogs; sometimes by licks on open sore.	2-6 weeks (10 days in head bites); may be as long as one year	Sporadic. Epizootics of rabies in wild animals such as wolves, bats, foxes, coyotes and skunks are potential reservoirs for rabies virus. Disease may spread to a number of domestic animals, including cats and cows, but canine rabies is mainly responsible for urban outbreaks. Head and neck bites cause more infections in man than bites on other parts of the human body.
Rocky Mountain Spotted Fever	Rickettsiae	Tick-borne.	3-10 days	The majority of cases occur in April and May, when the wood tick is prevalent. People in outdoor occupations are in greatest danger of being bitten by infected ticks. Control of ticks has been disappointing; personal care and immunization is the best insurance.
Dysentery (Shigellosis)	Bacteria	Fecal-oral, contaminated food, milk, water, carriers.	1-7 days	Disease is endemic only in areas where poor sanitary practices prevail; it may cause epidemics or sporadic outbreaks in the presence of local breakdown of sanitation. Most common in summer and in prisons, camps, and institutions; and in children. The reservoir is usually infected humans.

Signs and Symptoms	Prevention

Mild cough becomes violent and spasmodic. Coughing is followed by loud whooping sounds as the individual attempts to breathe. Disease usually of 6 weeks duration in 3 stages approximately 2 weeks each. *Catarrhal stage:* upper respiratory infection with increasingly intense non-productive cough and rhinorrhea; sometimes low-grade fever. *Spasmodic stage:* in 10 to 14 days cough becomes strangling and explosive, ending with characteristic whoop; thick, ropy mucus; vomiting; exhaustion; mental confusion. *Convalescent stage:* gradual decrease in severity of symptoms.

Immunization.

Plague appears in 3 forms: bubonic, septicemic, and pneumonic. Headache, dizziness, and thirst are early symptoms. High fever, restlessness, rapid breathing, fast pulse. Enlarged lymph nodes or buboes appear on second day. Pneumonic plague is marked by cyanosis, followed by convulsions and coma.

Immunizations should only be used when exposed to endemic areas.

Fever, headache, vomiting, malaise, sore throat, stiffness and pain in back, weakness, flaccid paralysis (in spinal type of disease). In bulbar type, respiratory paralysis, inability to swallow or talk clearly.

Immunization with all three types of vaccine.

Sense of apprehension, headache, vague sensory changes. Paralytic manifestations, in 2 or 3 days, first cause spasm on drinking. Delirium, convulsions, respiratory paralysis, death. Once symptoms appear, disease is usually 100% fatal.

Immunization given in the event of a bite by rabid animal or to persons in high risk occupations.

Disease resembles typhus, including the prodromal symptoms and sudden onset with headache, chills, prostration, and quickly rising fever. Marked muscle and joint pains and often bleeding from the nose. In untreated severe cases, fever ends late in the third week. The rash resembles that seen in early measles, which fades and is followed by lesions on ankles, wrists, legs, arms, chest.

Immunization.

Acute onset with frequent stools, diarrhea (frequently bloody and mucoid). Cramping in severe cases with fever. The disease is more severe in children because convulsions may occur. Bacteria invade mucous tissues and create abscesses.

Control depends almost entirely on sanitary measures, including surveillance of food handlers and water supplies.

Disease	Pathogen	How Transmitted	Incubation Period	Characteristics of Occurrence
Smallpox	Virus	Contact-inhalation. Virus-laden droplets or dusts are inhaled.	10-12 days	Infection is endemic and recurrent in some areas of Asia, Africa, South America, and the Middle East.
Tetanus	Bacteria	Usually, contamination of puncture or deep wounds.	4-12 days	This bacteria is found in the soil, but boiling is usually not sufficient to destroy. The disease is painful and fatality approaches 20%.
Tuberculosis	Bacteria	Contact-inhalation of droplets from infected person; milk from tuberculous cows.	2-10 weeks	Susceptibility is general; high in children under 3, lowest 3-12 years, relatively high remainder of life, overcrowding and malnutrition contribute to spread.
Typhoid/ Paratyphoid	Bacteria	Contaminated food and water spread through fecal or oral contamination.	10-21 days	Large epidemics of typhoid fever, once common, have been ended by modern water supply and sewage disposal and milk pasteurization. Remaining cases can be traced to contaminated food and to rare typhoid carriers. Man is the only reservoir. Paratyphoid fever is a closely related disease caused by certain other species of Salmonnellae. It is spread in the same manner as typhoid.
Typhus Fever (epidemic)	Rickettsiae	Louse-borne.	6-15 days	Epidemic disease in many African, Asian, and Eastern European countries. This disease is related to, but not identical with, endemic or murine typhus, a mild disease maintained in certain parts of the U.S. Typhus vaccine protects only against louse-borne typhus.

MUMPS

More than 16,000 children between the ages of five and ten get the mumps each year in the United States; complications among young children are usually mild or rare, but among young adults the mumps can result in sterility (in males), deafness, and juvenile-onset diabetes.

Adult males who have never had the mumps should be immunized to prevent the complication of sterility. Children should be given the vaccine at the age of fifteen months (often in combination with measles vaccine).

Signs and Symptoms	Prevention
Sudden onset with backache, headache, and vomiting, followed by eruption of pocks, which start as macules, become papules, then vesicles, finally pustules. Disease varies from mild to severe. Nine different grades of severity have been described, with mortality ranging from 0 to 100%.	Immunization is usually only recommended for those in high risk areas or those traveling into endemic areas. Routine immunization is no longer recommended.
Tightness in neck, general irritability, stiffness of muscles, inability to open mouth. Convulsions and cyanosis. Extensor spasms in which the head and heels are bent backward, and the body forward.	Immunization.
Malaise, lassitude, fatigue, fever, weight loss, hoarseness, cough, expectoration and hemorrhage from lungs. In some cases, the infection may spread to bones and kidneys.	Immunization for high risk persons, and pasteurization of milk.
Typhoid fever ranges in severity from a mild disease of 1-2 weeks' duration to a "fulminating," rapidly fatal illness. Usually malaise, headache and fever develop gradually. Anorexia, nausea, vomiting, constipation. Nosebleeds are common. Fever in untreated cases gradually rises to 102-104°F (delirium), with sweats and chills. Diarrhea. Paratyphoid has similar symptoms.	Immunization for those traveling into endemic areas. However, vaccine does not offer full protection.
After mild prodromal symptoms, such as fatigue and headache, the disease suddenly manifests itself with severe headache and bodywide pains; fever rises to 104°F and stays there until recovery. A rash usually appears on the fifth day on the back and chest, spreading to the abdomen and extremities, but usually not extending to the face, palms, and soles. Small hemorrhages in these lesions cause them to turn purplish in the second week. Stupor and coma foreshadow a fatal outcome. When typhus is contracted by immunized persons the symptoms and duration of the disease are greatly reduced.	Immunization for those traveling into endemic areas.

DIPHTHERIA, PERTUSSIS, AND TETANUS

Called the DPT shot, one immunization affords protection against all three diseases. Diphtheria can result in paralysis, heart failure, and death if it goes untreated; pertussis, better known as whooping cough, can lead to brain damage, lung collapse, and convulsions; tetanus, or lockjaw, claims almost half of its victims despite excellent medical treatment.

Given in a series of five shots, the vaccine should be first administered to children at the age of two months.

139

Adults can receive a separate tetanus shot if they are wounded five years or more after the DPT series ended or more than five years after they received a tetanus shot. Puncture wounds allow infected spores to enter the body, and all young adults and adults should receive tetanus shots if such a wound occurs after protection has lapsed.

SMALLPOX

Since it has been more than thirty years since smallpox has occurred in the United States and because October of 1977 saw the last case of smallpox anywhere in the world, the Public Health Service no longer recommends routine immunization of children.[26] However, you should be vaccinated against smallpox if you are traveling to a country that requires such a vaccination or if you are traveling to a country that has record of recent infection.

TYPHOID

Due to improving sanitation and other control measures, the number of typhoid cases has been steadily declining, and routine typhoid vaccination is no longer recommended in the United States. If you come into contact with a known typhoid carrier, if there is an outbreak of typhoid fever in the area where you live, or if you plan to travel to a country where typhoid fever is prevalent, you should be vaccinated. Vaccination is no longer recommended for areas that have been flooded or for children going to summer camps.

YELLOW FEVER

Yellow fever occurs today only in South America and Africa, and vaccination is recommended for persons over the age of six months who travel in areas where yellow fever still exists. (If you do require a vaccination for travel, you must receive it at a Yellow Fever Vaccination Center; such centers are listed with the World Health Organization.)

BUBONIC PLAGUE

Bubonic plague, a disease associated with wild rodents, occurs so rarely in the United States and elsewhere in most areas of the world that vaccination is no longer recommended unless you travel to Laos, Cambodia, or Vietnam, where the disease has reached epidemic proportions. Those whose work brings them into contact with wild rodents in South America, Africa, Asia, or the western United States should receive vaccinations, as should laboratory personnel who work with plague-infected rodents or plague organisms.

As long as you remain under a condition that may lead to infection, you should get a booster shot every six to twelve months.

VIRAL HEPATITIS

Persons living in households with hepatitis patients and persons who travel to tropical areas should be vaccinated with immune serum globulin (ISG) against hepatitis. The vaccination should only be taken if recommended by a physician.

INFLUENZA

Although influenza shots were recommended for the general public for two or three years during the mid-1970s, they are no longer recommended for most people, partly because flu viruses change their makeup from year to year and partly because there are so many different strains of flu virus.

Influenza vaccines are recommended for those who suffer serious consequences from the flu: children and adults of all ages who have chronic conditions such as diabetes, heart disease, kidney disease, chronic bronchitis, emphysema, asthma, or tuberculosis; adults over the age of sixty-five, since flu is often harmful to people in that age bracket and can lead to death; and those who are in extended-care facilities, where outbreaks may infect large numbers of people.

About every ten years there is a drastic change in the composition of the flu virus, and those who have built an immunity to previous strains of flu are infected, and thousands of deaths occur worldwide. During those times flu vaccinations are often administered to anyone who desires them.

RABIES

Only one to three cases of rabies are reported each year in the United States, but because the disease is almost always fatal, researchers continue in their efforts to further refine the rabies vaccine.

There is always a dilemma about how and if to treat a victim of a bite that may have been exposed to rabies because all forms of available treatment carry with them adverse side effects. In some cases the vaccines themselves have resulted in death. Factors that determine whether an individual should be vaccinated include the following:

- The species of the animal that bit: meat-eaters and bats are much more likely than other kinds of animals to be infected.
- The presence of rabies in the area.
- The circumstances of the bite incident: It the attack was unprovoked, the chances are greater that the animal was rabid.
- The vaccination status of the biting animal: It isn't likely that a housepet that has been vaccinated for rabies will carry and transmit the disease.
- The type of exposure: Scratches from a rabid animal or contamination of an open wound *can* result in rabies, but an animal bite is more likely to carry risk of infection.

Rabies vaccinations come in a series of twenty-four. Prompt cleansing and

tetanus immunization should follow all animal bites, and a physician will determine whether the rabies series should be started.[27]

SEXUALLY TRANSMITTED DISEASES

In any single year, approximately 8 to 10 million Americans have some kind of
venereal disease: gonorrhea, syphilis, genital herpes, trichomoniasis, or non-
gonococcal urethritis.* All of these diseases have one thing in common: They are
all spread through sexual contact.

Accordingly, those most affected by venereal diseases are those in the most
sexually active group—from fifteen to thirty years of age. Symptoms, complications, and treatment vary from disease to disease.

GONORRHEA

Gonorrhea accounts for approximately 2.7 million infections in this country
alone; worldwide, there are approximately 100 million cases, and the number is
rising. Gonorrhea has become the most common human bacterial infection.

Gonorrhea can almost always be traced to sexual contact with an infected
person; rarely is gonorrhea contracted from an inanimate object, such as soiled
clothing or toilet seats, because the gonococcus bacteria is extremely delicate and
survives very poorly outside the human body. The bacteria is especially prone to
die in open air or under significant changes of temperature.

Gonorrhea is the oldest and most well known sexually transmitted disease.

SITES OF INFECTION

While gonorrhea most commonly affects the genital area, it can settle in
other sites of the body as the disease progresses. Women commonly have rectal
infections, which can occur without participation in rectal intercourse. Rectal
gonorrhea is also extremely common among homosexual men.[28]

Gonorrheal infections of the throat are common among men and women
who engage in oral sexual activity.[29]

Gonorrhea that occurs at nongenital sites usually do not cause obvious
symptoms and often do not respond to the same antibiotics that are effective in

*The basis for this section taken from *Sexually Transmitted Diseases* (Bethesda, Md.: U.S.
Department of Health, Education and Welfare, National Institute of Allergy and Infectious Diseases,
Public Health Service, National Institutes of Health, 1977), DHEW publication no. (NIH) 76-909.

treatment of gonorrheal infections of the genitals. It is critical that the physician be informed of the full range of sexual activities so that treatment can be complete.[30]

SYMPTOMS
Symptoms typically first occur in the lining of the genital and urinary tracts.

In men painful urination and discharge from the tip of the penis is common. Most of the time symptoms appear about a week after sexual relations with an infected person; sometimes the symptoms take longer to appear, however, and at other times no symptoms at all appear in men. In infrequent cases the pus and discharge appear as soon as two days after exposure.

In women infection of the urethra and the cervix is usual. Many women never develop symptoms of gonorrhea; those who do frequently suffer vaginal discharge and painful urination. A newborn infant who passes through a mother's infected birth canal may acqure a potentially blinding infection of the eyes; as a preventive measure, physicians place silver nitrate or penicillin eye drops in the eyes of all infants immediately following birth.

TREATMENT
Treatment for gonorrhea consists of two injections of penicillin given simultaneously with probenecid, an oral tablet designed to increase the effectiveness of penicillin. Ampicillin, an oral medication similar in chemistry and pharmacology to penicillin, may also be used in treatment. Those allergic to penicillin and ampicillin may be given tetracycline or spectinomycin hydrochloride.

Once treatment is begun, symptoms begin to clear up quickly, and the individual may no longer be contagious in as soon a period as twenty-four hours. Some stay contagious for longer periods, however, and follow-up examinations are important.

It is critical to take all of the medication that is prescribed. Your symptoms may disappear within a day or two, and you may assume that you are better and quit taking medication. Even though symptoms may disappear, the infection will still remain; the entire course of antibiotics should be used. Since a certain dosage is required, you should never attempt self-treatment.

In gonorrhea, as in all other venereal infections, early treatment is essential to success in cure. Many venereal diseases can have severe complications if treatment is not begun immediately. If you have any reason to believe that you may have contracted a venereal disease, or if you notice symptoms that appear to be venereal in origin, you should seek medical attention immediately. Prompt medical help can help ensure a quick cure, can prevent complications, and can keep you from infecting others without knowing it.

PENICILLIN-RESISTANT GONORRHEA

A new strain of penicillin-resistant gonorrhea has been termed by the American Social Health Association as one of the most serious health threats to have arisen in a number of years. Due to mutation, some of the gonococcal bacteria have developed the ability to resist treatment by penicillin and other antibiotics. Instead, the new strain of gonococcus actually destroys penicillin.[31]

There *is* treatment available, but it requires a substitute drug—one that is approximately ten times the cost of penicillin and that takes much longer to cure the gonorrhea. In general, it is much more difficult to cure the new penicillin-resistant form of gonorrhea.[32]

The danger is that as the new strain of gonorrhea spreads, it may become resistant to new drugs formulated for treatment.[33]

COMPLICATIONS

When treatment is neglected or is insufficient, complications of gonorrhea can cause local tissue damage or more widespread damage through bacteria that enter the bloodstream and spread throughout the body.

In men, narrowing or blockage of the urethra is a common complication. Spread of the infection to the tubes that carry sperm from the testes can result in sterility. In severe cases it is necessary to stretch the urethra mechanically so that urination is possible.

In women the bacteria may spread up the reproductive tract and cause a painful infection known as pelvic inflammatory disease. A serious infection of the uterus, fallopian tubes, and ovaries, pelvic inflammatory disease results in permanent abdominal pain (even after the condition is cured), large pus-filled abscesses, and sterility. Each time pelvic inflammatory disease occurs, it increases the risk of developing future attacks. Fever, nausea, vomiting, abnormal vaginal bleeding, and pain during intercourse are some of the symptoms of this disease. Women who are pregnant when they contract gonorrhea experience high rates of spontaneous abortion, prematurity, and stillbirth.

The most common complication of gonorrhea in both sexes is arthritis; the affliction comes on suddenly with chills, fever, and joint pains beginning one to four weeks after the first infection. The knees, wrists, and ankles are involved most frequently.

Much less often inflammation of the brain or the lining of the heart occurs as a complication of gonorrhea; in rare cases gonococci invade the blood and cause serious complications.

Even when complications occur, a case of gonorrhea does not provide immunity against future cases; recurrences following therapy are rare, so most cases of infection that occur after therapy are new infections.

SYPHILIS

Though syphilis is not as widespread as gonorrhea, it is one of the most devastating of the sexually transmitted diseases if it is left untreated. Partly because of diligent efforts to identify and treat possible carriers, syphilis is much less frequent than gonorrhea in North America. Most cases of syphilis in the United States now occur among men homosexuals.[34] Estimates place the number at about half a million.

Like gonorrhea, syphilis is spread by direct intimate contact with the lesions of someone in the infectious stages of the disease. Also like the gonococcus, the syphilis bacterium is fragile and is thus unlikely to survive outside the body long enough to permit contraction from inanimate objects.

SYMPTOMS AND COURSE OF DISEASE
Syphilis progresses in three distinct stages:

Primary syphilis. The first of the stages, primary syphilis, is characterized by a hard, painless sore, or chancre, which appears anywhere on the body where the bacteria entered—usually on the genitals, lips, or anus—usually from three to four weeks after exposure. Swelling in the small lymph glands surrounding the chancre usually develops, especially in the groin area. Because the chancre is painless, it may go unnoticed—especially if it develops in the vagina or, as is the case with many homosexual men, in the rectum. The most common sites for the chancre are on the tip of the penis and in the vagina or on the cervix. The chancre will spontaneously disappear, usually within six weeks.

Secondary syphilis. After the chancre disappears, the infected person is symptom-free until about ten to fourteen weeks after exposure to the infection, when symptoms of secondary syphilis develop if the disease was not treated in its primary stage. Most common is a skin rash that can appear anywhere on the body anywhere from two to twelve weeks after the chancre disappears. It may be only on the hands and feet, or it may cover the entire body. It is generally accompanied by fatigue, fever, loss of hair, headaches, muscle aches, lesions in the mouth, and swelling of the lymph glands in several areas.

The symptoms of secondary syphilis disappear even without treatment within two years—a fact that leads may victims erroneously to think that the infection has cleared up. The bacteria, however, remain in the system and will cause serious problems years later.

It is only during the first two stages of syphilis that the person is contagious and can pass the infection on to others. The exception to the rule is a pregnant woman who, for a much longer period, can transmit the disease to her unborn child.

Latent syphilis. If secondary syphilis goes untreated, it will develop into the third and final stage of syphilis, a stage of undetermined length. The bacteria are dormant for a period that may last anywhere from one to thirty years; when it reactivates, it brings with it possible blindness, heart disease, paralysis, insanity, other mental illness, and death.

TREATMENT

As with gonorrhea, treatment consists of penicillin injections given during a single visit to the doctor's office; the infected person is generally no longer contagious within twenty-four hours after treatment. Those who are allergic to penicillin are given tetracycline, erythromycin, or cephaloridine. If early treatment is initiated, all signs of syphilis can be eradicated from the blood in six months to two years. In all stages of syphilis the treatment will cure the disease, but the organ damage that accompanies the final stage cannot be reversed.

COMPLICATIONS

A woman who is infected with syphilis during pregnancy can pass syphilis on to her unborn infant after about sixteen to eighteen weeks of pregnancy. If the mother is treated before that time in the pregnancy, the disease will not be passed on; if she is treated after that time but before the birth, the child will be cured. If there is no evidence of reinfection during later pregnancies, there is no reason to re-treat the mother with each new pregnancy.

Syphilis that is not treated during pregnancy results in a child who is born with congenital syphilis—a disease occurring during the first two years of life and involving deformities of the bones, skin, teeth, eyes, and other parts of the nervous system. Care must be taken in handling a child with early congenital syphilis, because the moist lesions are infectious.

As with gonorrhea, one syphilis infection does not provide immunity to future attacks.

GENITAL HERPES

Gonorrhea and syphilis are both caused by a bacteria, but other agents can also be transmitted sexually—including a virus that results in a condition called genital herpes and caused by the herpes simplex virus.

One form of the virus—type 1—is best known as the cause of cold sores and fever blisters that afflict many individuals from time to time. The familiar lesions of type-1 herpes simplex virus can occur anywhere on the body above the waist, and are most common around the mouth.

Another kind of herpes simplex virus—type 2—causes lesions to develop below the waist, most commonly on the genitals. While genital herpes is not as serious as gonorrhea or syphilis, herpes infections are quite painful and disabling; like fever blisters, they tend to recur.

There are about 300,000 cases of genital herpes in the United States today.

The herpes virus is present in the fluid of the skin lesions and in some of the bodily secretions (including saliva and urine) of the infected person; it is spread by close contact—but not necessarily intercourse. Primary lesions tend to appear in those from the ages of fifteen to thirty, but recurring lesions (those that recur after the initial infection) may appear any time later in life.

SYMPTOMS

Genital herpes begins with a primary infection; the virus goes into hiding in certain parts of the nerve cells and reemerges spontaneously in response to sexual contact, menstruation, other infections, emotional stress, and nonspecific conditions. The primary genital herpes infection is usually more disabling than later recurrences.

Two to twelve days after exposure to the virus a small sore or cluster of sores appears at the site of exposure—usually on the penis or in the urethra in men and on the cervix, in the vagina, or on the external genital area of women. The sore may be quite painful with local swelling, and there may be fever and other general body symptoms of infection.

The symptoms of primary infection disappear in two to three weeks, and the virus may remain hidden for years before recurring.

The blisters that accompany primary infection may appear on the back, buttocks, hands, or other areas that have been infected. The blisters usually break open shortly after they form, especially in women, and the resulting open sores are extremely painful.

During recurrence the only involvement is generally with the local lesion, which usually occurs in the same place as did the primary lesion. Some involve pain, but sores in the cervix, upper vagina, urethra, or prostate produce no symptoms at all. Recurrences are usually healed within one to two weeks.

TREATMENT

Antibiotics, which are effective against bacterial infections, have no use in the treatment of viral infections; genital herpes treatment usually centers on use of pain-relieving ointments, good genital hygiene, loose-fitting underwear, repeated smallpox vaccinations, dye accompanied by light exposure, and antiviral vaccines (still in the experimental stages).

To minimize the discomfort of genital herpes and to hasten healing of the sores, you should keep the infected area clean and dry; wash the infected area three or four times a day with a mild soap and water, and rinse thoroughly. Make sure the area is completely dry. You can add talcum powder or cornstarch to your underwear if you perspire heavily. Wear loose-fitting cotton underwear to prevent the spread of infection and to help keep the area dry; women should not wear

147

panty hose until the sores have healed, and neither men nor women should wear nylon underwear. Don't use ointments or creams unless they have been prescribed by your doctor.

COMPLICATIONS

As with other forms of venereal disease, the main complication of genital herpes is for the pregnant woman and the unborn baby. Genital herpes infection during pregnancy causes a high rate of stillbirth and spontaneous abortion. Many babies are born prematurely.

The baby's contact with genital herpes sores as it passes through the birth canal can result in a crippling or fatal form of meningitis: inflammation of the tissues and membranes surrounding the brain and spinal cord. When genital herpes is diagnosed in a pregnant woman, the baby is usually delivered by cesarean section in order to avoid its exposure to the virus.

Less frequent complications of genital herpes include narrowing of the urethra or inflammation of the nerves. Scientists are currently researching the link between genital herpes and cancer of the cervix.

NONGONOCOCCAL URETHRITIS (NGU)

Also known as nonspecific urethritis, NGU is probably about twice as common as gonorrhea and is caused by sexual contact—not by strain and stress, too much spicy food, allergy, alcohol, or too much sex. Most of the NGU cases that are diagnosed are in men, but women are frequently infected, too.

About half of the cases of NGU are caused by a rare bacterium called *Chlamydia;* the exact cause of the other half is unknown.

SYMPTOMS

The symptoms of NGU in the male are the same as gonorrheal symptoms—discharge from the penis and painful urination—but they are usually milder than with gonorrhea. Some men who are infected have no symptoms at all. As with gonorrhea, women frequently have no symptoms; in some, irregular menstrual periods, genital irritation, vaginal discharge, or pain in the lower abdomen are present.

COMPLICATIONS

The complications of NGU are generally serious and long-term. It can cause serious inflammation in the testicles and is the major cause of inflammatory pelvic diseases in women.

TREATMENT

Tetracycline is the best antibiotic to use in the treatment of NGU; erythromycin is a perferred alternative. Oral antibiotics must be taken four times a day for at least a week to clear up the infection. You must abstain from sexual intercourse until the infection has completely cleared up.

MINIMIZING RISKS

Of course, the best way to reduce your risk of developing a venereal disease is to abstain from sexual relations completely. If you do not choose that course of action, there are other things you can do to minimize your risks, although none is completely effective.

You should limit the number of sexual partners you have. Two people who have sexual intercourse only with each other will never get venereal disease unless one of them already had it.

Choose sexual partners who also limit their number of partners; your risk of developing venereal disease is lower if you choose sexual partners who also limit their number of partners.

Be choosy when it comes to sexual partners; avoid having sex with anyone who has sores or rashes of any kind on the genitals, a general body rash, or a discharge of any kind from the penis or vagina.

Immediately after having sexual intercourse, urinate and then wash the genital area completely with soap and water.

Proper use of a condom—placing the condom on the penis as soon as foreplay begins and removing it as soon as intercourse is finished—can help protect the man and the woman from venereal disease. The condom should completely cover the penis and should not have any tears or leaks in it; it should be new, and should be kept in its original foil packet until use (condoms that are kept in pockets or near the body are prone to deteriorate as a result of body heat and perspiration). The man should withdraw as soon as he can after he ejaculates to prevent the penis from softening inside the vagina; the condom often slips off if the penis is allowed to soften. You should dispose of the condom immediately, since it may contain infected matter.

Some protection for the woman can be obtained from using a vaginal contraceptive foam.

REFERENCES

[1]*Arthritis: The Basic Facts* (New York: Arthritis Foundation, 1976), preface.

[2]Ibid.

[3]Ibid., p. 6.

149

[4]John Talbott, "Coping with Gout," *Drug Therapy,* May 1978, pp. 99–102.

[5]*Arthritis: The Basic Facts,* p. 20.

[6]*How to Cope with Arthritis* (Washington, D.C.: U.S. Department of Health, Education and Welfare, Public Health Service, National Institutes of Health, 1976), DHEW publication no. (NIH) 76-1092, pp. 12–14.

[7]*The Facts About Diabetes* (New York: American Diabetes Association, 1966), p. 1.

[8]Ibid., pp. 4–5.

[9]Glen R. Schiraldi, *Diabetes! What Now?* (Provo, Utah: Utah Valley Hospital and Glen R. Schiraldi, 1977), pp. 10–11.

[10]*Pollen Allergy* (Bethesda, Md.: U.S. Department of Health, Education and Welfare, Public Health Service, National Institutes of Health, National Institute of Allergy and Infectious Diseases, 1976), DHEW publication no. (NIH) 75-493, pp. 4–5.

[11]*U.S. News and World Report,* January 1973, pp. 40–41.

[12]Irwin Ross, "Allergy," *Consumer's Digest,* March–April 1977, p. 14.

[13]"What's Good for Hay Fever?" *Consumer Reports,* June 1977, p. 342.

[14]"Allergic? You *Can* Be Helped," *Changing Times,* January 1976, p. 35.

[15]"Allergies," in *The Health Letter,* 8, no. 6 (1976), published by Communications, Inc., San Antonio, Texas; edited by Lawrence E. Lamb.

[16]Alvin Silverstein and Virginia B. Silverstein, *Allergies* (Philadelphia: J. B. Lippincott Company, 1977), p. 69.

[17]"Allergic? You *Can* Be Helped," p. 35.

[18]William Cole, ed., *Digestive Diseases* (Bethesda, Md.: U.S. Department of Health, Education and Welfare, Public Health Service, National Institutes of Health, 1977), DHEW publication no. (NIH) 76-1073, p. ii.

[19]Shirley Morrison and Carolyn Arnold, *Communicable Diseases,* 9th ed. (Philadelphia: F. A. Davis Company, 1969), p. 4.

[20]Ibid., p. 5.

[21]J. Imperato Pascal, *The Treatment and Control of Infectious Diseases in Man* (Springfield, Ill.: Charles C Thomas, Publisher, 1974), p. 4.

[22]Gaylord W. Anderson, Margret Arnstein, and Mary Lester, *Communicable Disease Control,* 4th ed. (New York: Macmillan, Inc., 1962), p. 26.

[23]Ibid., p. 27.

[24]"Important! Get the Kids the Shots They Need," *Changing Times,* May 1979, p. 45.

[25]Ibid., p. 46.

[26]Faye Peterson, "Vaccine Recommendations," *FDA Consumer,* July–August 1978, p. 14.

[27]Ibid., p. 13.

[28]H. Hunter Handsfield, "What You Need to Know About VD," *Drug Therapy,* June 1979, p. 104.

[29]Ibid.

[30]Ibid.

[31]*Some Questions and Answers About Penicillin-Resistant Gonorrhea* (Palo Alto, Calif.: American Social Health Association, 1977).

[32]Ibid., p. 53.

[33]Ibid., p. 53.

[34]Handsfield, "What You Need to Know," p. 105.

CONSUMER HEALTH

As a consumer in today's health market, you have probably contributed to the $700 million spent on aspirin in the United States annually;[1] you are probably one of the 179 million Americans covered by health insurance;[2] and, most likely, the hours you spend in front of your television expose you to low doses of radiation.[3] And as a consumer in today's health market, you probably wonder if there's something better than aspirin, if you really have enough (or too much) health insurance, what you can do about television set radiation—and how you can solve a myriad of health-consumer problems critical to your well-being.

Issues vital to you as a health consumer run the gamut from how to find a good doctor to how to read a prescription to how the environment affects your health.

THE ENVIRONMENT

Russell E. Train, former administrator of the U.S. Environmental Protection Agency, maintains that many of the chronic diseases we are plagued with today are a result of environmental factors—what we eat, where we live and work, our habits, and our life-styles.[4] Because we have learned to acknowledge the role of the environment in maintaining health, there is no way we can responsibly avoid the challenges of improving and correcting environmental defects.

AIR POLLUTION

Air pollution results from chemicals being regurgitated into the air from smoke-stacks, automobile exhaust pipes, and fires of any source. At its best, it causes or worsens such conditions as bronchial asthma, pulmonary emphysema, and bronchitis. At its worst, it results in death.[5]

Air pollution isn't a recent problem: During the last half of the nineteenth century citizen groups in London clamored for cleaner air, but their protests were drowned by the goal of industrialization at any cost. Since the dawn of the Industrial Revolution people in many communities have endured air standards that would not be considered permissible today.[6] Nor does air pollution only plague those in highly urbanized areas; agricultural fires and coal waste fires are major contributors to air pollution today.

POLLUTANTS

The greatest source of air pollution is transportation—particularly the automobile. By weight, transportation accounts for almost half of all air pollutants. Several major pollutants (including carbon monoxide, nitrogen oxides, and hydrocarbons) are introduced by transportation.

Primary pollutants include the following:

Carbon monoxide. Lighter than air, carbon monoxide is an odorless, colorless, poisonous gas that results from incomplete burning of carbons in fuels. Carbon dioxide, a natural element in the atmosphere, is produced instead where there is enough oxygen to ensure complete combustion.

Almost two-thirds of the carbon monoxides in the air come from internal combustion engines, the overwhelming bulk of them in automobiles and other gasoline-powered motor vehicles.

Sulfur oxides. Electric utilities and industrial plants are the principal producers of sulfur oxides—corrosive, acrid, poisonous gases that result when fuel that contains sulfur is burned. (The major fuels of utilities and industries are coal and oil, both of which contain sulfur.) About 60 percent of the sulfur oxides in the air are the result of burning coal; 14 percent are caused by burning oil, and 22 percent by industrial processes that use sulfur.

Two-thirds of the sulfur oxides are emitted in urban areas, where population and industry are concentrated; seven industrial states in the Northeast account for almost half of the total sulfur oxides emitted in the United States. Large industrial plants, smelters, and power plants in rural areas may also be culprits. (A single large industrial plant may throw off as much as several hundred thousand tons of sulfur oxides in a single year.)

Government agencies and research organizations have sought to reduce sulfur oxide pollution by removing sulfur from fuels entirely, by removing sulfur oxides from combustion gases, and by switching to low-sulfur fuels.

Particulate matter. Particulates—literally particles of waste material in the air—come in solid and liquid form and in a variety of sizes. Some particles are so large that they are visible as soot; others are so small that they can only be detected through an electron microscope. Most particulate matter is a result of stationary fuel combustion and industrial processes; forest fires and other miscellaneous sources account for about 34 percent of the particulate matter in the air. When particulate matter is very small, it can remain in the air for long periods of time and can be transported long distances by the wind.

There are several established techniques that help control particulate matter. Complete removal of particulate matter from a boiler stack or waste air stream is impossible—or at least technically and economically difficult—but larger particles can be removed by methods such as centrifugal separation, electrostatic precipitation, filtering, and washing.

Hydrocarbons. Like carbon monoxide, hydrocarbons result when fuel is not completely burned; unlike carbon monoxide, however, hydrocarbons are normally found in the atmosphere at low concentrations, and, at those low concentrations, are not toxic. They are, however, harmful in larger concentrations: They are responsible for forming photochemical smog.

More than half of the hydrocarbons produced each year come from transportation sources—mostly gasoline-fueled vehicles. More than half is found in urban areas, mainly because of the higher concentration of automobiles.

Nitrogen oxides. When fuel is burned at extremely high temperatures, as it is in many industries, nitrogen oxides are produced; when combined with sunlight and hydrocarbons, nitrogen oxides form a complex variety of secondary pollutants called photochemical oxidants. When combined with the solid and liquid particulate matter found in the air, photochemical oxidants also produce smog, with its thick haze and offensive odor.

The control of nitrogen oxides, of course, consists of carefully controlling temperature in the burning of industrial and other fuels. Controlling the nitrogen oxides in automobile exhaust is more difficult, because the methods used to control other pollutants often increase the concentration of nitrogen oxides.

All of these elements of air pollution are influenced by a variety of factors, including weather, wind speed, density of atmosphere, and topography (areas located in basins or valleys or backed up against mountains are natural traps for pollutants in the air).

EFFECTS OF AIR POLLUTION

The most important effect of air pollution is on human health. Severe episodes of air pollution in such cities as New York and London have resulted in a dramatic increase in serious and life-threatening health problems that can be directly traced to pollutants in the air.

We have come to expect many of the results of air pollution, and many are familiar to us as we wipe at our stinging eyes and roll up our windows when caught in traffic. Other effects are not as widespread, and some afflictions occur only among those who are already susceptible by virtue of a preexisting condition or illness.

Current clinical studies, industrial research, laboratory experiments, and studies from industrial accidents are supplying scientists with information that confirms the role of air pollutants in the following diseases:

Nonspecific upper respiratory disease. The effects of air pollution on the respiratory tract mainly affect the cilia, tiny hairlike cells that line the airways and that act to propel mucus—and the germs and dirt that are caught in it—out of the respiratory tract and that act to protect the underlying cells of the respiratory tract. Air pollutants have been demonstrated to slow down and even stop the action of the cilia, and in severe cases they can even cause a loss of cilia. As a result, underlying cells become exposed to the dirt and pollutants contained in the mucus; in extreme cases pollutants can even destroy the several layers of cells beneath the cilia. Pollutants have also been shown to cause the production of increased or thickened mucus, to induce swelling or excessive growth of the cells that line the airways, and to cause a constriction of the airways.

As a result of all these effects, the common cold—usually believed to be caused by a virus—may in some cases be indirectly caused by pollutants in the air. While pollutants cannot cause a cold per se, they can produce coldlike symptoms and can increase a person's susceptibility to colds. The coldlike symptoms that result from air pollution (and that are often confused with colds) are called acute nonspecific upper respiratory disease.

Chronic airway resistance. The narrowing of the airways in the presence of an irritant is referred to as chronic airway resistance. Such restriction can be either a temporary or, as in many cases, a permanent condition. Studies have shown that no single pollutant is responsible but that most kinds of pollutants result in chronic airway resistance due to inflammation of the bronchioles and injury to the trachea and bronchial tubules.

Bronchial asthma. Asthma is actually an allergic reaction, and bronchial asthma consists of an abnormal reaction of the airways to the air that is breathed. Asthma can result from any of a number of agents, among them pollutants in the air. Breathing is restricted by widespread narrowing of the bronchioles, by mus-

155

cle spasm, by swelling of the mucous membrane, or by a thickening and increase of the mucous secretions. Though it is chronic, asthma comes in short periods called attacks, and the respiratory tract returns to a normal state following each attack.

Chronic bronchitis. Chronic bronchitis—a recurrent and lasting cough—is caused by pollution and by a number of other factors, including cigarette smoking, heart disease, lung infection, and lung cancer. When other factors are absent, physicians generally attribute sole responsibility to pollutants in the air. Not only do air pollutants *cause* chronic bronchitis, but they cause preexisting cases of the disease to worsen markedly.

In studies completed in Great Britain and the United States common pollutants were shown to diminish or stop the production of mucus and were shown to interfere severely with the lung's ability to fight off bacteria—both leading contributors to chronic bronchitis. Defined as a cough that brings up phlegm (mucus) on most days for three months of two successive years, chronic bronchitis can also lead to other chronic and recurrent bronchial infections.

Pulmonary emphysema. Pulmonary emphysema is closely linked to chronic bronchitis: It can occur simultaneously with or as a resultant follow-up of chronic bronchitis.

In cases of emphysema the tiny air spaces at the ends of the bronchioles— the *alveoli*—undergo a breakdown of cell walls; as the emphysema progresses, the alveoli become enlarged, lose their resiliency, and eventually disintegrate— all permanent tissue changes. These permanent tissue changes in the lungs result in shortness of breath, and emphysema in its most serious stages is often a secondary cause of death.

Whatever the original causes of emphysema, it is certain that air pollution aggravates and worsens the condition; in many cases asthma and chronic bronchitis accompany the emphysema, leading to a multiple-disease condition. A strong relationship exists between the air pollution index and the number and severity of emphysema cases; that relationship increases when cigarette smoking is also present.

Lung cancer. Originating in the bronchial mucous membrane, lung cancer is characterized by abnormal, disorderly new cell growth; it is usually fatal.

Like emphysema, lung cancer cannot be attributed to any one cause, but recent scientific findings indicate that both cigarette smoking and atmospheric contaminants play a major role in the development of lung cancer. Some scientists believe that the ability of pollution to destroy or inhibit ciliary action and growth may be the key in development of lung cancer. Statistical studies reveal that there is a much higher incidence of lung cancer among those living in areas of dense air pollution than among those living in cleaner air, all other factors being similar or identical.

New correlations have been found between influenza and lung cancer. In one experiment mice were infected with a flu virus; survivors had little higher rate of lung cancer than control mice. The survivors of the influenza were then exposed to air conditions that mimicked smog; the incidence of lung cancer was increased sharply.

Heart disease. Chronic respiratory diseases—common accompaniments to air pollution—place undue stress on the heart and the surrounding blood vessels, leading to various kinds of heart disease. There are other reasons that air pollution results in heart disease: The loss of oxygen that results from respiratory disease forces the heart to pump harder and faster in order to circulate sufficient oxygen through the body; carbon monoxide, a common element of polluted air, reduces the oxygen content of the blood, placing stress on the heart; and those with preexisting heart conditions are endangered by even mild air pollution.

Other health effects. In addition to specific diseases that result from air pollution, chemical elements in the air cause dizziness, headaches, blurred vision, impaired reaction time, reduced fertility, lethargy, susceptibility to influenza, lead poisoning, eye irritations, and arteriosclerosis. Some scientists have hypothesized that air pollution contributes to premature aging.

In severe cases it results in death.

WATER POLLUTION

What about the quality of the water available to us all? As a rule, the most bacteria-laden water is found in rural areas, where water gets little or no treatment. Urban dwellers, on the other hand, trade in bacteria for extensive chlorine treatment, which, when combined with organic material in the water, sometimes produces cancer-causing agents.

Residents of rural areas (or urban area residents, if they are interested) can determine the quality of the water available to them by calling the state health department or by arranging for a private laboratory to test the water samples from the area. Unfortunately, because of the newness of tests and because of the expense involved in obtaining equipment, few of America's 240,000 public water systems and few of the millions of private wells in the United States have been tested for carcinogens—cancer-causing agents that recent research indicates may be abundant in some water supplies.

Where is the biggest danger involving carcinogens in the water? Amarillo, Texas; Annandale, Virginia; Brownsville, Texas; Camden, Arkansas; Cape Girardeau, Missouri; Charleston, South Carolina; Cheyenne, Wyoming; Columbus, Ohio; Concord, California; Hackensack, New Jersey; Houston, Texas; Huntington, West Virginia; Huron, South Dakota; Ilwaco, Washington; Jackson, Mississippi; Louisville, Kentucky; Melbourne, Florida; Miami, Florida; Montgomery, Alabama; New Orleans, Louisiana; Newport, Rhode Island; Norfolk, Virginia; Oklahoma City, Oklahoma; Omaha, Nebraska; Passaic Valley, New Jersey; Phoenix, Arizona; Santa Fe, New Mexico; Tampa, Florida; Terrebonne Parish, Louisiana; Topeka, Kansas; Washington, D.C.; Waterbury, Connecticut; and Waterford Township, New York, all exceed the federal limits placed on carcinogens (calculated on a parts-per-billion basis).[7]

Water supplies in Baton Rouge, Louisiana; Boston, Massachusetts; Fresno, California; Greenville, Mississippi; Jacksonville, Florida; Madison, Wisconsin; Portland, Maine; Provo, Utah; Pueblo, Colorado; Rockford, Illinois; Spokane, Washington; Tacoma, Washington; and Whiting, Indiana, have been found to contain the least traces of carcinogens in public water sources tested in the United States.

It's important to note, however, that both clean and polluted (or carcinogenic) water can be found in the same location. For instance, wells in Long Island, most of which are less than 100 feet deep, are contaminated with high-level cancer-causing agents. Long Island's deep wells, however—those extending to 400 feet—yield clean water free of the carcinogens.

Pollutants and carcinogens in America's water supplies gave rise to dozens of home water filter companies in the latter half of the 1970s, with Americans purchasing 2 million of the gadgets each year in an attempt to trap chemicals and pollutants before they escape the tap. According to the Environmental Protection Agency and the Water Quality Association, most of the filters sold fit on an incoming water line, on the counter, under the sink, or in the tap; some filter all the water used in the household, while others allow a bypass for water that is not used for cooking or drinking. A few companies offer handheld models that operate similar to a coffee filter. Costing anywhere in the range from ten to several hundred dollars, the filters are effective in trapping naturally occurring minerals (such as calcium), but EPA officials stress that no standard unit can remove suspected cancer-causing agents from the water.[8]

Water pollution—"the presence in water of any substance that impairs any of water's legitimate uses"[9]—results in health problems in addition to cancer, including outbreaks of disease caused by contaminated drinking water (in the decade from 1961 to 1970, there were 130 officially recorded disease outbreaks, some of them involving as many as 16,000 people in individual episodes[10]). Damage to the central nervous system results from eating fish or fowl contaminated by mercury. Other pollutants—including pesticides, asbestos, iron ore, Mirex, and insecticides—have found their way into many of the nation's major water supplies. Microorganisms found in some water supplies have bred bacteria and viruses that cause cholera, typhoid, hepatitis, salmonellosis, and gastroenteritis.

There are other ill effects of water pollution, too—including the destruction of wildlife and the loss of valuable recreation areas. Phosphates washed down drains ends up in lakes, where overgrowth of vegetation chokes and clogs the lake systems. Every year millions of gallons of sewage are deposited in lakes and bays, destroying fish and other animal life and rendering some areas (such as Michigan's Lake Erie) useless for recreation.

The problem of water pollution has reached enormous proportions. Every year more than 400 million tons of pollutants enter the waters of the United States[11] from dairy plants (53 billion gallons of waste water and 200 million pounds of solids),[12] hospitals (170,000 tons of pathological waste),[13] chemical warfare agent treatment (70,000 tons of residual salt),[14] municipal sewer systems (40 billion gallons of effluent daily),[15] industry (125 billion gallons daily),[16] agriculture (50 billion gallons daily),[17] and rainfall (which washes 44 million tons of sulfates, nitrates, bicarbonates, and chlorides out of the atmosphere each year).[18]

Current efforts at control are centered on sewage treatment facilities, restrictions on industry, and legislation designed to prevent further pollution of water supplies, especially those used for drinking water. One of the most damaging and perplexing pollution problems is fairly recent in its origin: the major oil and petroleum spills and pollution resulting from shipment of oil in tankers and from offshore drilling for petroleum and oil reserves. With emphasis being placed on alternative methods of finding solutions to the energy problem (including coal mining in the United States), the threat of petroleum pollution may be somewhat decreased.

MICROWAVES

Microwaves—extremely high-frequency radio waves—are known to most for their role in microwave cooking, but microwave technology is also used in aviation, weather forecasting, communications (70 percent of all the long-distance telephone networks in the United States are operated by microwave), cable television, closed-circuit communications, pest control, and intercontinental communications via satellite.[19]

Though microwaves are capable of causing injury if used directly, damage has been infrequent; generally the only form of microwave that is used directly is the microwave oven, and most are safe when used according to manufacturer's instructions. (Some may interfere with heart pacemakers when used in close proximity.) Federal standards require that all ovens manufactured after 1971 not emit radiation above specified levels, and that each oven be equipped with at least two independently operating safety interlocks to shut off radiation as the doors are opened; each oven manufactured after 1971 must also bear a manufacturer's label stating compliance with federal regulations.

There's a great deal you can do to ensure the safety of a microwave oven. Study the manufacturer's recommended operating procedures carefully, and follow all instructions pertaining to operation and maintenance. Examine the oven carefully for signs of freight damage; if you see anything even slightly suspect, don't use the oven until a qualified repairman has inspected it for safety.

Never operate the oven while it's empty. Never insert objects through the door grill or around the door seal. Never tamper with or inactivate the oven safety interlocks.

Switch the oven off before you open the door. While you are operating the oven, stay at least an arm's length away from the front of the oven. Clean the oven cavity, the door, and the seals frequently with water and mild detergent (*do not* use scouring pads, abrasives, or steel wool on a microwave oven).

Have the oven serviced regularly by a qualified repairman who can check for signs of wear, damage, or tampering.[20]

PROTECTING YOURSELF
AS A HEALTH CONSUMER

Because of pollutants in our environment and because of habits and life-style patterns, we as Americans are becoming increasingly aware of our responsibility as health consumers. As we are learning to take more of the responsibility for our own health, our reliance on members of the medical profession has decreased and condensed to only those services we cannot provide for ourselves.

As a health consumer, you have the right to choose the health professionals you want to deal with and to question diagnostic tests and examination procedures when you don't understand them or when you feel they are unnecessary.

HOW TO CHOOSE
A DOCTOR

One of the most important considerations you can make concerning health care professionals is that made in choosing a doctor. As a patient, you have certain rights:[21]

The right to choose a doctor. You have a right to quality care, and you have the right to choose the doctor that will afford you the best care. You have the right to check a doctor's background and training, and you have the right to contact your local or county medical society for the names of accredited physicians (these societies will not recommend one doctor over another, but they will give you the names of as many accredited physicians as you desire).

The right to change doctors. Too many patients feel that they have to stay with one doctor because he or she has their medical history on file and has treated previous conditions. Though a doctor who knows your medical history is at a distinct advantage, you should never feel you have to stay with a doctor who is not satisfying you.

The right to privacy. Your medical condition, any information concerning it, and your remarks while in the doctor's office should be protected with the utmost care. No one who is not involved directly in your health care should have access to any information about your medical condition or history unless you give specific written permission. (Even health insurance companies must have your written permission—your signature on a health insurance form—before they can obtain information concerning your treatment from your doctor.) A doctor who violates this rule of privacy in any way is subject to strict penalties from the American Medical Association.

The right to full information. You have the right to know as much—or as little—as you want to know about your condition, your treatment, the results of tests, the purpose of tests, the kind of medication your doctor is prescribing, and possible side effects of that medication. You not only have the right to ask questions, but you have the right to complete, truthful answers. If your doctor refuses to tell you the information you want to know, you have the right to go elsewhere for medical treatment.

The right to know medical costs and fees. You have the right to ask exactly what your medical care will cost before you submit to treatment. You should never agree to treatment, tests, or other procedures until you know how much they will cost. Your doctor should be willing to discuss his or her fees and should be willing to reveal any prices involved.

The right to a second opinion. Especially important in cases of catastrophic illness requiring extensive treatment or in cases of surgery is the right to go to a second doctor for his opinion before submitting to any treatment. Unless yours is a life-or-death situation, you should have ample time to obtain at least one additional opinion.

In cases of surgery it is required that you obtain a surgeon's opinion in addition to your family doctor's opinion; getting a third opinion (from another qualified surgeon) is always wise. One prominent West Coast surgeon estimated that obtaining second and third opinions reduces the amount of unnecessary surgery as much as 60 percent.

When you seek a second opinion, make sure that the surgeon is qualified: Just because a doctor performs surgery does not mean that he or she is certified for surgery; almost half of the operations performed in the United States each

161

year are performed by doctors who are not certified by the American Specialty Board. To determine a doctor's qualifications, read the certificates hanging on the office wall; there should be one there from one of ten American Specialty Boards. The letters FACS following a doctor's name indicate a designation by the Fellows of the American College of Surgeons.

Most patients make two big mistakes in choosing a doctor: They choose the doctor on the basis of his or her personality, and they choose the specialist to fit an ailment they *think* they have (a method that is nothing more than self-referral).[22] Those patients couldn't be more wrong. Though a pleasing personality makes the patient-doctor relationship better, it is certainly not the best basis for choosing a doctor. Instead of choosing a specialist, it is best to choose a doctor who is concerned with you as a whole person—not simply as a bundle of nerves or a collection of bones. You should have one primary doctor—a general practitioner—who can see you *each time* you have a complaint and who, on the basis of your complaint and your medical history, can then refer you to a specialist if necessary.

Three general types of doctors fit under the general practitioner category:

Family physician or general practitioner. Sometimes difficult to find in dense urban areas, a family physician or general practitioner is trained to take care of general medical problems that occur from birth to death. In most cases he or she can handle diagnosis and treatment; in some cases referral to a specialist must be made. The family physician or general practitioner is ideal for most people, single or married, especially those in their twenties and thirties with young children; he or she treats all family members and keeps a detailed medical history on file.

The internist. Since middle age brings on a number of chronic medical conditions (such as heart disease, ulcer, diverticulitis, diabetes, or hypertension), the internist—a doctor specializing in internal medicine—is the best bet for those middle-aged or older, whose children are grown.

The obstetrician. Though an obstetrician is a specialist in pregnancy and childbirth, he or she can serve as a primary doctor for a woman in her childbearing years, since many medical problems are related to childbearing. If you expect to use an obstetrician as your primary doctor, make sure the physician is aware of your expectations; talk them over carefully with the doctor. Some may express discomfort in trying to fulfill that role, and you should take the cue to find another primary physician.

An important consideration in choosing a physician is the kind of practice the physician has. A doctor who works independently (without partnership or association in a clinic) affords you the best in a personal relationship. Frequently such a doctor comes to know your medical history so well that he or she can diagnose some simple problems by phone. Whenever you make an appointment, you are assured of seeing *that* doctor. If you choose to go with a solo doctor, make sure that he or she makes adequate arrangements for another doctor to cover while ill or on vacation.

A doctor who works as one of a group of four or five family physicians or general practitioners (generally associated with a clinic) offers several advantages. The doctor you regularly see has the benefit of being able to call on an associate to confirm a diagnosis or to help solve a puzzling problem. In dealing with a group of doctors, you are generally able to see a doctor any time of the day or night for emergency treatment, since at least one doctor is generally available. In some clinics you are able to choose one doctor to treat you most, if not all, of the time; in other clinics you must take an appointment with any doctor that is available at the time. If you want to develop a personal relationship with one doctor and if you do not like to switch doctors, you should either go with an independent doctor or you should be sure of the practices of the clinic you choose.

A large multispecialty group of doctors works much like the group of four or five general practitioners except that the multispecialty group contains physicians in all areas of specialty. The normal practice is that you choose one physician in the group—usually an internist—as your regular doctor, and you make appointments with that person when you need to see a doctor. He or she may then refer you to any of the other specialists in the group (or, sometimes, outside it). One advantage of a large multispecialty group is that they usually work in a clinic, where specialized diagnostic tools and machinery are available (patients rarely have to go to the hospital for diagnosis, a practice that means savings on health care costs). The disadvantage of large multispecialty groups is that a primary doctor may have the tendency to refer patients to specialists within the group almost as a matter of course—at a great expense to the patient. Some patients who desire a close interpersonal relationship with the physician are unable to find it in the large multispecialty group.

The type of medical care available to you will depend on the community you live in; rural areas generally have only family practitioners, whereas urban areas have mostly specialists. If you live in the suburbs, you usually have a wide choice.

To locate a physician that will serve you best, begin by calling your county medical society and asking for the names of two or three family physicians, general practitioners, or family internists in your neighborhood. Ask the same question to the local medical exchange answering service and the administrator's office of your local hospital. When you call, describe the kind of medical service you require (your age, how many children you have, the type of physician you've had in the past, or any special problems you may have). The medical association or the medical exchange will probably select names at random from a rotating list, but the hospital administrator's office should be able to give you the names of physicians who might better suit your personal needs.

Seek the advice of people in the community whom you respect and who have lived in the community for a number of years (a good person to ask is a banker, a school administrator, a lawyer, or a clergyman). Then ask a neighbor. Add any names you get to your list. Especially important are the names of physicians who might have helped others successfully through a long-term illness.

Check with related professionals, such as dentists, nurses, and pharmacists. A nurse is a particularly good source of advice: He or she will have had the opportunity of working with many of the doctors in the hospital and will have observed firsthand the level of patient care each affords. If you are moving to a new community and need to locate a doctor there, ask your current doctor for a recommendation.

Find out which physicians in your community have served as chiefs of departments at the local hospitals or who have headed up community organizations for better medical care. These are usually well respected by their colleagues.

If you already have a specialist—such as an ophthalmologist or a dermatologist—ask which primary physician he or she personally uses.

Look at the list you have compiled. If two or three names keep coming up again and again, those doctors will probably be best to begin with in your search for a good doctor. Make an appointment for a routine matter—a sore throat or a physical for college. Then talk to the doctor as you are being examined, and look for the following:[23]

The doctor should have obtained a complete medical history from you on your first visit and should have asked a number of detailed questions about your own medical past and about your family's medical history.

Even if you are consulting the doctor for a specific complaint, you should have been given a pretty complete physical examination at your first visit. If you are a woman, you should have been given a breast examination, a pelvic examination, and a rectal examination. The doctor should have arranged for a Pap smear. If you are a man, you should have been given a rectal examination.

The doctor should have spent enough time with you to answer your questions and to satisfy your concerns. He or she should have given you a complete diagnosis and should have been willing to answer any questions you have concerning it. He or she should have treated you as a participant in your health care instead of a mindless victim.

If you are pleased with the initial visit and decide to go back to the same doctor, watch for these characteristics:

The doctor should keep medical records, taking notes as you discuss your problems; he or she should consult those records each time you come in for an examination.

At least once every five years the doctor should obtain certain basic laboratory tests, such as blood and urine analyses. The doctor should voluntarily discuss the results of those tests with you.

Periodically, the doctor should measure your blood pressure and should discuss the results with you. At your yearly exam (or in some cases, more frequently) the doctor should arrange for an electrocardiogram to test your heart function; again, he or she should voluntarily discuss the results.

The doctor should be concerned about your personal habits—your diet, your sleeping patterns, whether you smoke or drink, how much you exercise—and should ask you questions concerning your life-style and habits. He or she should be willing to give you advice concerning any aspect of your life-style you ask about.

Does the doctor involve you in patient education by making available brochures, pamphlets, or books that concern your special problems? He or she should provide you with explanatory material that you can take home with you if you want further information about your individual medical problems.

The doctor should spend an adequate amount of time with you to answer your questions. You should feel free to ask any question—even if it sounds foolish to you. If you are embarrassed to ask a foolish question, then you don't have the kind of rapport you should have and you should probably seek another doctor.

If the doctor orders diagnostic tests to be performed, he or she should willingly describe what each test diagnoses, how each test works, and why each test is being ordered for you. He or she should also be willing to reveal the cost to you and to consult you concerning cost before ordering the tests.

If the doctor prescribes medication, he or she should be willing to explain what the medication does, what its possible side effects are, and why the medication will be helpful for you. If you ask, he or she should be willing to list the contents of the prescription for you on a separate piece of paper so you can keep it at home. If possible, the doctor should be willing to prescribe generic drugs as a way to save costs; in cases where a generic drug would be ineffective, he or she should be willing to explain why.

The doctor should arrange for someone to take over while he or she is taking a day off or is on vacation. If the doctor is not willing to be disturbed at night, he or she should arrange for a competent doctor to take calls during the evenings.

If they are really necessary, the doctor should be willing to make house calls. (Keep in mind that the vast majority of house calls are not necessary.)

The doctor should be willing to talk to you on the telephone during office hours to answer simple questions that will save you the trip to the doctor's office.

(The doctor should not, however, be expected to make a diagnosis over the telephone.) If a doctor is busy with a patient, he or she should be willing to return your call within a reasonable length of time. A doctor who is never available by phone is usually not genuinely concerned with the patients.

When making a diagnosis, the doctor should explain it fully to you and should be willing to answer all questions you have concerning it. Where there is a viable alternative concerning treatment, the doctor should let you help make the decision.

The doctor should be involved in activities to keep up to date concerning medical research and recent findings. Ask if he or she attends meetings and seminars, reads medical journals, or does other things to continue his or her medical education. The doctor should belong to one or more medical societies; if a specialist, he or she should be board certified and should take steps to keep current on medical advances.

To make the most of your visit to the doctor, be prepared ahead of time to do your part. Be able to tell the doctor the following:[24]

The history of your present illness. Before you arrive at the doctor's office, sit down and figure out exactly when your throat started to feel raw. What happened first? Did you get nauseated before your headache started, or did the headache precede the nausea? If you get flustered when you go to the doctor, write down your symptoms and take the paper with you. Be prepared to tell the whole truth—even if the questions or answers are embarrassing.

When describing your present illness—the complaint that brought you to the doctor's office in the first place—you need to tell the doctor everything you can about *all* of your symptoms. Just as important, you should tell the doctor what you think might be wrong. Someone with a headache that has lasted for weeks may fear he or she has a brain tumor; expressing that fear to the doctor may help alleviate some of the tension that has increased the severity of the headache.

Don't keep the doctor playing guessing games. Answer questions truthfully, and express your fears and doubts fully. Your doctor shouldn't be shocked or upset by any disclosures you make; if he or she does react that way, you should get a new doctor. Remember, the doctor is legally bound to keep everything you divulge in confidence; you needn't fear that others will find out what you have told the doctor.

Your past medical history. On the first visit, the doctor will want to know your complete medical history—especially serious diseases you have had (and, most particularly, those of a chronic nature, such as diabetes, high blood pressure, mental illness, ulcers, or migraine headaches). Tell the doctor anything you can about your handicaps, too: Be sure to mention that you are nearsighted or that you only have one kidney.

If your doctor does not ask you for the information, tell him voluntarily about any dental work or dental X rays you may have had. In some cases, infection from decaying teeth may enter the bloodstream and travel to other parts of the body.

You should especially be familiar with the medical history concerning the complaint you have now. If you have been suffering with severe headaches for months, it would be important for the doctor to know that you also had a long-term bout with severe headaches several years ago. Details from a previous illness may help the doctor make a more accurate diagnosis of a present illness.

Your family's medical history. This may take a bit of research before you go to the doctor's office, but it will be well to your advantage if you can tell the doctor the medical history of your parents, brothers, and sisters. Certain diseases—among them cancer, heart disease, diabetes, allergy, gout, and certain kinds of mental illness—tend to be hereditary (in some, the tendency to develop the disease is hereditary, even though the disease itself is not). If a doctor knows that your father died of cancer of the colon, he or she will be more thorough in checking out a complaint of rectal bleeding and may order diagnostic tests to check for early cancer. If both your parents have hypertension, your doctor will probably want to check your blood pressure each time you come in for an exam and may give you advice concerning your diet and your life-style that will help you avoid developing hypertension.

Your psychological history. An accurate psychological history is important in assessing your physical condition. Many diseases are at least partially caused by psychological conditions; it's important that you tell the doctor how you feel about things, how your moods affect you, whether you have been depressed. If your relationship with someone is causing you a great deal of anxiety, you should tell your doctor. If your fears of failing a particularly difficult class are interfering with your ability to study for other classes, confide your fears in your doctor. He or she may be able to discuss ways of overcoming your problems and will probably be able to find explanations for vague physical symptoms that are bothering you.

Your environmental history. The water you drink, the air you breathe, what you do for fun, how many hours you study each night, how many cups of coffee you drink in the morning, how many meals a day you eat, whether you walk or drive to work—all these are part of your environmental makeup, and can adversely or positively affect your health and well-being. Even factors as remote as your sexual life or your driving habits can influence your health, and your doctor should have an accurate assessment of all habits and life-styles.

Once having taken down your medical history, the doctor will examine you and, hopefully, make a diagnosis. You need to play an active part in physician-patient communication to ensure that you make the most out of your visit to the doctor. Keep the following in mind:[25]

Write down any questions you have before you get to the doctor's office; then, in the confusion of the exam, you won't forget them. Don't feel that you have to confine yourself to questions about your current problem: You may want to ask the doctor something about sexual relations, a symptom you had last year, or for help in improving your diet. If you were constipated after taking the antibiotic the doctor gave you for last year's ear infection, discuss it and ask why if it bothers you.

If you don't understand what the doctor is saying, say so. The doctor has spent years getting a medical education and may take for granted some of the basic medical jargon. Or, he or she may have seen hundreds of patients with complaints just like yours and may inadvertently skip over some basic explanations. Your doctor might think you know what a cyst is or why cutting down on salt will help reduce your blood pressure. If you don't, ask for an explanation; you shouldn't be embarrassed to have to ask for clarification, and if your doctor embarrasses you, find another doctor.

If the doctor decides to give you a shot, find out what it will and won't do. If you stepped on a nail playing touch football in the field behind the dorm and the doctor prescribes a tetanus shot, find out how long the shot will be effective and exactly what protection it affords. If you are suffering from earache, headache, and sore throat and the doctor gives you a penicillin shot, find out which symptoms the shot should alleviate and in what period of time; then, in two weeks, if the sore throat is still bothering you, you will know that further treatment is still needed.

If the doctor prescribes drugs, find out as much as you can about them. Write down the information as the doctor gives it to you: How long should you take the drug, and how often? What should the drug do for you? What adverse side effects might you suffer? How will the drug interact with other drugs you are taking? Will the drug make you drowsy? Can you drive or operate machinery while taking the drug? Can you drink alcohol while you are on the program of drug treatment? Will the drug make you nervous? (When you get to the pharmacy, ask the pharmacist to include the patient package insert with the drug; it explains many things your physician may not think to tell you.)

Write down all the instructions the doctor gives you—including those that indicate restrictions on your activity. You may think you have a great memory, but a week from now you may not remember exactly how many glasses of water you were supposed to drink every day.

If the doctor diagnoses a long-term or serious illness, do some homework. The public library should have information that will help you learn about the disease and that will help you ask intelligent questions the next time you go for a checkup. As you read, make notes of questions you need to ask your doctor.

Whatever your diagnosis, find out what's ahead. If it's mononucleosis, find out how long you'll probably be needing bed rest. Find out how soon you can expect to resume normal activity. Find out what the normal pattern of symptoms is and find out under what circumstances you should come back for another checkup.

There are things you can do with your doctor to cut down on your medical bill.[26] If you have a regular primary doctor, talk to him or her by phone before you come to the office. If your doctor is well acquainted with your medical history and if the problem is minor, he or she can probably diagnose over the phone and save the office charges. If you become ill at night or on a holiday, call your primary doctor instead of going to the hospital emergency room; office charges are always less than emergency room fees, and many emergency room physicians will simply call your own doctor anyway or will treat you temporarily and instruct you to call your doctor the next day.

Discuss the cost of medical care with your doctor. If you are on a tight budget and your ability to pay is limited, be frank in explaining your limitations. A doctor who realizes that you are on a very tight budget may refer you to free services, may lower his or her own fee, or may decide against expensive procedures if there's a choice. He or she will probably prescribe generic drugs when possible in order to help you save money at the pharmacy.

As discussed earlier, write down your questions and your list of symptoms in advance so you can be direct and brief; many doctors bill you according to the amount of time you spend in the office.

Be in tune with your own body and serve as your own early-warning system. You can usually tell when something is wrong: If your bowel movements turn gray, you may have something wrong with your liver or gallbladder; if your urine is brown or black, you may have bleeding somewhere in your urinary tract. Pay attention to symptoms and seek medical attention promptly. Ignoring problems will not make them go away, and the longer you delay, the more likely you will be to require extensive medical treatment—at a much higher cost than simpler procedures.

As a last resort, keep track of your medical expenses for tax purposes. You can deduct expenses such as medical insurance premiums, payments to doctors, payments for hospital services and laboratory tests, payments for psychiatric care, payments for medicines and drugs and prescribed vitamins, the cost of a special food that your doctor prescribes for your illness, payment for transportation that makes it possible for you to receive medical care (keep track of mileage if you use your own car), meals and lodging that you need as part of your medical care, the cost of special equipment that is installed in your home or car as a result

169

of your physical condition, and payments for artificial limbs, teeth, eyeglasses, hearing aids, crutches, and other equipment.[27]

HOW TO CHOOSE
A HOSPITAL

In some areas of the country and in some communities you may not be able to make a choice among hospitals: One may serve an area of several communities or of an entire county. In other cases you may choose a physician that will only work in one of the hospitals in your community. At the end of the last decade there were more than 7,000 hospitals in the United States; major surgery costs averaged $10,000 in representative metropolitan areas.[28] Where you do have a choice, you should consult with your doctor about which hospitals he has privileges with, and you should make sure you are getting the most for your money by checking the following:[29]

Is the hospital accredited? Only 4,800 of the nation's 7,000 hospitals are accredited by the Joint Commission on Accreditation of Hospitals (a nonprofit organization composed of medical associations that serves to set optimal—rather than minimal—standards for patient care). Every year thirty-five survey teams review almost three thousand hospitals, and those that have fallen below optimum standard have their accreditations made probational. Hospitals that are accredited display their credentials in the lobby; if you don't see a certificate of accreditation in the lobby, ask the hospital administration or write to the Joint Commission on Accreditation of Hospitals, 875 North Michigan Avenue, Chicago, Illinois 60611.

Is the hospital general or special? For most illnesses you are better off in a general hospital, where costs are lower and the staff is able to handle a wide variety of problems. General hospitals usually offer a complete range of services, and in some general hospitals (especially those affiliated with universities) departments have been organized to handle various specialties. Though special hospitals are generally more expensive, they are recommended for patients who need specialized treatment generally unavailable in a general hospital. For example, a cancer victim may get more specialized treatment at Memorial Hospital in New York City, or an asthma victim may need the specialized treatment available at National Jewish Hospital in Denver.

Rural hospitals tend to be staffed by general practitioners or family physicians, and patients needing extensive or specialized care may need to be transferred to a larger general hospital in an urban area.

Is it a teaching hospital? Teaching hospitals are those that have approved programs for teaching resident physicians; many are affiliated with universities and serve as the practical arm of the university's medical school. Some community-owned hospitals have one or more teaching programs that are operated in cooperation with a nearby medical school. There are about 400 major teaching hospitals in the United States.

If you are seriously ill, you should seek a teaching hospital, where specialized care and facilities are available to you. The latest equipment and the best-trained physicians are generally found at teaching hospitals. And some forms of treatment or therapy are available only at teaching hospitals, where careful monitoring of the experimental therapy can be undertaken.

There are some disadvantages to teaching hospitals. As a rule, they tend to be cold and impersonal. The patient—especially the patient who is critically ill or who has an unusual disease—is often subjected to pawing and prodding by strings of residents and student nurses. Because student residents and nurses learn from authentic patient conditions, the patient's stay may turn out to be longer, and the chances of infection are sometimes increased.

Remember that in most teaching hospitals the primary goal is teaching; the secondary goal is patient care. In many cases research goals come ahead of patient care, too.

How many beds are in the hospital? As a rule the quality of patient care is better in a hospital that has more than 100 beds than in a hospital that has fewer than 100 beds; larger hospitals generally have better equipment, physicians who are better trained in current procedures, and special units (such as coronary care units and intensive care units). In many small rural hospitals with fewer than 100 beds it is sometimes difficult even to find a physician on duty when an emergency comes up; the physician who is on call may take up to fifteen minutes to arrive at the hospital—and in some cases, fifteen minutes can spell the difference between life and death.

There are some small hospitals (with 25 to 50 beds) that offer excellent service. Small hospitals that are accredited and that have one or more specialists on the hospital staff, facilities for coronary and intensive care, and an adequate number of nurses trained in coronary resuscitation and intensive care procedures are generally excellent hospitals, despite their small size.

Who operates the hospital? Hospitals fall under several types of ownership: community (nonprofit), religious groups (usually nonprofit), private ownership (profit), and university (usually profit). A hospital is eligible for accreditation if it meets optimum health-care standards, regardless of ownership.

In general, hospitals run for profit (usually those that are privately owned) try harder to please patients and doctors because their facilities are more expensive and because they are dependent on patients and doctors to turn a profit.

Hospitals run for profit generally offer fewer special services and the quality of health care is slightly below that of hospitals run by nonprofit organizations.

Warning signs. As a final criterion in choosing a hospital, you should be aware of certain signs that signal problems that might eventually result in substandard patient care. Watch out for

- Financial problems (as reported by the local media, or as revealed in financial reports)
- Internal disputes, such as strife between the doctors and the administrative staff (such disputes are commonly reported by the media)
- Unrest or strikes by hospital employees
- Signs of disorder as you walk through the hospital
- Staff doctors who have had disciplinary actions taken against them by the state licensing board or the state medical society

Once you have been in a particular hospital, you can further assess its quality of health care by noting several characteristics:[30]

Was there one primary nurse coordinating your care? Just as your primary physician coordinates your care with the other physician specialists while you are in the hospital, an efficient and quality hospital will have one primary nurse coordinating your care with all nurses on all shifts.

Was there some amount of tender loving care? Nurse shortages across the country have created conditions in hospitals that have resulted in a minimizing of personal care for patients, but some things should still be expected. When you ring for a nurse, one should answer within one to two minutes; a delay longer than two minutes is indicative of an inadequately staffed hospital. A nurse who cannot deal with your problem on his or her own should immediately call your physician for instructions. Most important, a nurse should check you periodically whether or not you have called for help. Such periodic checking is especially critical for patients who have been sedated.

What was the food like? Hospitals aren't meant to compete with first-class hotels, but you should still expect certain standards as far as the food is concerned. Menus should be well planned, and you should be offered a variety to choose from. Hot food should be served hot, and cold food cold—not lukewarm. If you are in the hospital for an extended period of time, the hospital staff should be willing to provide meals to those who stay with you for a small extra charge.

How was the housekeeping? You have a right to expect the utmost in cleanliness and comfort from the hospital. Stringent cleaning is necessary to prevent the risk of contamination or infection. Floors, window ledges, bathrooms, and general room areas should be thoroughly cleaned daily; utensils, pitchers, and bedpans should be washed out regularly throughout the day and should be changed from day to day. If you have a chance to inspect areas outside your room, look at the storerooms, closets, and the space behind emergency exit doors: If these are immaculate, the rest of the hospital probably is, too.

Is the physical structure of the hospital run down? Even the most rigorous cleaning will not correct peeling paint, exposed pipes, worn linoleum, and other structural defects. Hospitals should be kept in good repair year round. The best hospital is the one built with room on reserve that can be used to meet the hospital's expanding needs.

Is the financial status of the hospital sound? A hospital that is inadequately financed cannot maintain enough personnel, nor can it keep abreast of current developments in equipment and technique. Some hospitals have been on the verge of bankruptcy because their overzealous expansion was not backed by adequate financing. If you have reason to believe that a nonprofit hospital is suffering financially (if there didn't seem to be enough nurses, for instance), you can obtain a financial statement upon request to the hospital administrator.

SAVING MONEY IN THE HOSPITAL

Just as there are things you can do to cut down on your doctor bill, there are things you can do to cut down on the cost of hospitalization:[31]

Discuss your schedule ahead of time. Don't be admitted on a Friday if the hospital can't run laboratory tests on Saturdays and Sundays. Wasted days in the hospital still have to be paid for, even though you do nothing but lie in bed all day. Ask your doctor to coordinate with the hospital staff so that your time in the hospital is well utilized.

Have tests done ahead of time. If your tests can be performed outside the hospital before you are admitted, have them done at a local clinic. Clinic charges for tests are almost always lower than what the hospital charges. Then, too, you won't be paying for a hospital room while the tests are being conducted. Make sure your insurance pays for tests at clinics.

Ask for a ward or semiprivate room. While almost all hospitals have semiprivate rooms available, some will put you in a private room without asking your preference. Private rooms always cost more; a ward is the least expensive way to stay in the hospital.

Pass on air conditioning. If the admissions desk gives you a choice, choose a non-air-conditioned room. It will be less expensive, and air conditioning is not beneficial to healing and recovery.

Bring your own medication. Some hospitals will not allow you to bring your own pills, but if you can, check with your doctor to see what kind of medication you'll be needing, and get it ahead of time from your pharmacy. Medication is *always* more expensive in the hospital: a single aspirin will cost you fifty cents or more.

Don't take more drugs than you have to. Drugs in the hospital are expensive, and if you take more than you really need, you run the danger of suffering adverse side effects. Complications can result, and your hospital stay may be longer as a result. Find out what drugs you are taking, what they are designed to do, and what side effects they have. Then, when you really don't need that medication anymore, tell the nurse and have her contact your doctor.

Try to cut down on lab tests. Many tests, of course, are necessary, but some are done just to satisfy the doctor's curiosity or to assist in research (this is a particular danger in teaching hospitals). Tell your doctor ahead of time that you are on a budget and that you don't want any unnecessary tests run. Then make sure your hospital bill is itemized so you can justify what you are spending on tests.

If the hospital wants to run tests that were run earlier in the doctor's office, speak out. Refuse to have duplicate tests run unless there is a critical need for them (for instance, a duplicate test may be necessary if the hospital feels your condition has changed or if several doctors question the accuracy of the test).

Move around as soon as possible. The sooner you can get out of bed and start doing things for yourself, the sooner you will recover and be able to leave the hospital.

Avoid frills. Whenever you have a choice, take the no-frills plan. Some hospitals reduce the cost of health care for patients who can make their own beds, eat meals in the cafeteria, and perform other tasks for themselves; in some cases, the reduction is as great as 40 percent.

Don't stay in the hospital longer than you have to. Make sure that you know ahead of time what the discharge hours are and how far ahead of time the papers have to be signed; make sure you and your doctor agree on the discharge time and date. It is a waste of money to have to pay for another day just because your doctor didn't get the papers signed before noon.

Donate blood. If you will need to use blood during your stay in the hospital (during surgery or transfusion, for instance), donate blood ahead of time to pay for the blood you use. If your illness prevents your donating the blood yourself, arrange for a friend or a family member to donate it to the hospital in your name.

You might want to consider donating to the American Red Cross or the American Association of Blood Banks on a regular basis so that you and your family members will have a supply of blood on hand without charge when you need it.

Ask to be an outpatient. Sometimes your doctor will hospitalize you simply because it's more convenient for him. But unless you have to be hospitalized, you can save the cost of the hospital room by reporting to the hospital for tests and treatment during the day and then going home at night. Even many minor surgical procedures can be performed on an outpatient basis, with you reporting to the hospital for the surgery and then coming back several times to be checked.

Be treated at home. Depending on the nature of your condition, it may be cheaper to hire a nurse to come to your home to administer medication and perform other necessary duties. A visiting nurse can stop in several times a day and check your condition for your doctor.

Don't jump the gun on delivery. If your labor pains are slow and mild, wait awhile before checking into the hospital (unless, of course, your doctor expects complications and has ordered you to report at first sign of labor). Many hospitals begin their billing day at midnight, and you can save a whole day's cost by staying at home until your labor pains are more steady.

Check your hospital bill. If your hospital doesn't automatically provide an itemized bill, insist on one. Go over each charge carefully, and make sure you understand each one. If you have a dispute, bring it up and get it settled.

A final note on getting at the truth when you are a patient in a hospital: You are allowed to see your chart, according to law. Insist that hospital personnel let you see your chart and that they answer any questions you have concerning your condition. Prepare a list of questions to ask, and insist on answers.

DIAGNOSTIC TESTS

Like any other test, a medical test is designed to give information. Before any treatment can be carried out, a physician needs to know what, if anything, is wrong with the patient; this information is not always apparent from external signs or symptoms, and the physician may need to resort to a myriad of diagnostic tests to confirm suspicions or establish a firm diagnosis.[32]

You may have had diagnostic tests in the past, or may have them in the future, from a physician who is reluctant or unable to explain the procedure fully to you. There are several reasons for this:[33]

Because of constant advances in medical science, there is now a bewildering variety of diagnostic tests available to physicians. The physician who orders the test may know what it is for and what it tells him, but he may not know how it is performed, either because he has never seen it done or because it is so new that he is unfamiliar with the procedure. Physicians who order an upper GI series to diagnose a patient's suspected ulcer know full well what the test will reveal, but unless they've had an upper GI series themselves, they probably won't be able to tell the patient what one is like or what the procedure is.

Even when physicians do know the procedure for a diagnostic test, it is difficult for them to put themselves in the patient's place and anticipate what the patient's fears and concerns are. For example, a carotid arteriograms, where dye is injected into the carotid artery and travels to the brain to provide a picture of blood vessels in the brain, is generally frightening for a patient. A physician who sees many of the tests performed each year has come to accept them as commonplace and probably doesn't realize that the patient is afraid.

If the physician does not know the procedure for the test, the patient must rely on the laboratory technician for an explanation. Unfortunately, the lab technician is usually on a tight schedule, unable to spend more time than necessary with any one patient; he or she does not see the patient until the laboratory test is scheduled. In certain kinds of tests the technician does not see the patient at all.

Though some physicians know the procedures and are aware of the patient's apprehensions, many are reluctant to describe the procedure fully for fear of upsetting the patient further. Patients, however, have the right to be informed of the risks and discomforts of any diagnostic procedure, and you should insist on that right when you undergo any kind of diagnostic test.

X-RAY EXAMINATION

Probably the most valuable and the most widely used tool for diagnosis is the X ray—high-energy electromagnetic impulses that cannot be seen or felt as they pass through the body.[34] In extremely high doses X rays are capable of severely damaging or destroying human tissue (such high doses are used in treatment of some kinds of cancer to kill cancer cells); the low doses required for most diagnostic tests will not damage normal tissue unless certain precautions are not taken or unless a patient receives them too frequently.[35]

More than 240 million examinations each year use X rays as a diagnostic tool for doctors and dentists in the United States.[36] The most common diagnostic tests are chest and dental X rays.

Though the benefits of diagnostic X rays outweigh the disadvantages, recent findings indicate that overexposure to X-ray radiation may trigger serious disease or tissue destruction, including cancer. As an X ray passes through the body, some of the radiation is absorbed; more is absorbed by the dense body parts. The radiation, which is instantly dissipated into other forms of energy, can result in damage or destruction of cells from the transfer of energy. Most such damage is repaired by natural body processes, but some damaged cells can remain and cause serious problems as long as thirty years after exposure to the X-ray treatment or diagnosis.

You can take measures to protect yourself against the potential harms of X-ray diagnosis by doing the following:[37]

Keep accurate records of each X ray that you have—the type of X ray, what it was taken for, the name of the dentist or physician who gave you the X ray, and the date. Record the location of the facility where you received the X ray so that you can obtain the X rays if necessary.

Whenever your physician or dentist orders an X ray, ask for an explanation of why it is necessary. If you are not satisfied with the reason, tell him or her that you feel it is unnecessary. Find out if there is an alternate diagnostic method that will work as well. Be sure to mention if you have had similar X-ray tests performed before.

If you are changing communities or physicians, ask for your X rays. Some doctors or hospitals will release your X-ray file to you, and such files should be given to your new physician; they may prevent the need for further diagnostic tests using X ray.

Chest X ray screening programs for the diagnosis of tuberculosis are no longer recommended. If your employer requires that you be tested for tuberculosis prior to accepting employment, ask the doctor to give you a tuberculin skin test instead of a chest X ray.

Dental X rays are no longer recommended on a regular basis; they should only be used in specific instances to diagnose a suspected problem the dentist cannot diagnose in any other way. The American Dental Association has ruled that dental X rays should not be a standard part of every dental examination.

If they do not interfere with the diagnostic procedure, insist on a lead shield to be placed around your reproductive organs if you are having X rays of the lower stomach, lower back, abdomen, or any area near the reproductive organs. In addition to causing sterility in some rare cases, exposure to X ray may cause genetic damage in the chromosomes, which is then passed on to subsequent generations. Because the male's reproductive organs are located outside the body, it is particularly critical that a man request a gonadal shield if he is to receive X rays of the abdomen or lower back. It is less critical for a woman, but it would also be prudent for her to request a shield.

If you are a woman and have any suspicion that you might be pregnant, tell your doctor before he or she orders diagnostic X rays. Because X rays are damaging to a fetus, you should not receive them during pregnancy unless they are vital to saving your life. Even if you do not think you are pregnant, you should limit X-ray exposure to the first fourteen days of the menstrual cycle in order to prevent exposure to a fetus you may be unaware of.

Never demand an X ray if your doctor seems reluctant. Some doctors have resorted to unnecessary X ray to protect themselves in case of malpractice cases being leveled against them. You should avoid all unnecessary X rays, but you should realize that they are essential in some cases for accurate diagnosis.

SPECIAL-RISK GROUP

If you had X-ray treatments involving your head or neck as a child or young adult, you are now a member of a special-risk group and should contact your physician immediately to arrange for an examination of your thyroid gland. Those who were exposed to X rays in the treatment of ringworm of the scalp, enlargement of the thymus gland, deafness due to lymphoid tissue around the Eustachian tubes, enlargement of the tonsils or adenoids, or acne run a higher than normal risk of developing tumors of the thyroid gland any time from five to thirty years from the time of exposure.[38]

Fortunately, most of the tumors are benign and slow-growing; even when they are cancerous (malignant), they remain confined to the neck area for long periods of time. If discovered early, they can be successfully treated.

If you think you might have been exposed to X rays in such a course of treatment, contact your physician immediately and ask that your throat and neck be examined; then follow up with regular examinations every one to two years. (It is important to be examined even if you do not feel a lump.)

The examination, in which the physician feels the thyroid gland for any indication of swelling or a lump, is painless and takes only a few minutes. If your physician does find a tumor, remember that most tumors are *not* cancerous and respond successfully to simple treatment.

COMMON DIAGNOSTIC TESTS

Though there are hundreds of diagnostic tests available to physicians, the three most common are blood chemistry, urinalysis, and hematology—simple, quick tests using the blood and urine to reveal the general condition of the body and the presence of abnormality or infection.

BLOOD TESTS

In most cases only a few drops of blood need to be drawn to complete blood tests; the normal procedure is to prick the fingertip and extract a few drops of blood onto a prepared slide.

The first test run is the CBC—complete blood count. After diluting the drop of blood on the slide, the laboratory technician looks through the microscope and literally counts the blood cells by counting the number in a small marked area of the slide and calculating the total number based on that subtotal. Technicians count both red cells and white cells.[39]

In addition to counting cells, the technician notes the size and shape of the various blood cells. Abnormally large red cells, for example, appear in rare types of anemia; in other kinds of anemia the red cells may be pear-shaped or saddle-shaped, or may have a tail.

Too many red cells signals a condition where the body attempts to over-compensate for inadequate oxygen by producing more red blood cells; victims of congenital heart disease, or such respiratory disorders as emphysema, or of high-altitude living may overproduce red blood cells. Too few red blood cells signals anemia, inability of the bone marrow to produce red blood cells, or chronic blood loss due to internal bleeding somewhere in the body.

Too many white blood cells signal infection somewhere in the body. Leukemia also causes an increase in the number of white blood cells, and the cells are abnormal in appearance in cases of leukemia.

In addition to a count and assessment of blood cell appearance, blood tests are used to diagnose a number of diseases or abnormal conditions; blood chemistry tests determine the following:

- *Sugar (glucose)*—A blood glucose level that is too low may indicate that there is too much insulin being produced in the pancreas, that carbohydrates may not be absorbed, or that liver disease is present. A high blood glucose level may indicate the presence of diabetes or some other glandular disorder.

- *Protein*—High levels of protein in the blood may indicate the presence of some serious illness. Chronic liver, kidney, or gastrointestinal diseases may be indicated by low blood protein levels.

- *Nitrogen*—If the kidneys are not functioning properly, nitrogen levels in the blood may be high. Low levels may mean the presence of liver disease.

- *Calcium*—A high calcium level may result from an overactive parathyroid gland (this may also cause other serious bodily disturbances). When calcium levels are too low, it may be an indication of a parathyroid gland that is not functioning up to capacity, or it may mean that there is a vitamin D deficiency which can lead to malabsorption of calcium.

- *Cholesterol*—Low cholesterol levels can mean that the thyroid gland is oversecreting, that fats are not being properly absorbed in the intestines, or that other intestinal diseases may be present. High colesterol may be the result of a hereditary disorder so that fats are metabolized improperly, or it may be the result of overconsumption of saturated fats—each of which may signal potential heart and/or artery diseases.

- *Phosphate alkaline*—A high phosphate alkaline level may indicate that there is a bone fracture or injury or a liver injury.

- *Bilirubin*—When the bilirubin level is high, the bile ducts may be obstructed, or there may be jaundice (produced by liver disease) or abnormal destruction of blood cells.

- *Uric acid*—Kidney stones, kidney disease or malfunction, or gout can produce high uric acid levels.

Hematology tests, also run on a blood sample, determine the number of cells, their shape, and the percentage of red and white cells that comprise the bloodstream.

URINE TESTS

If the doctor can tell so much by testing your blood, why is it a general practice to have the urine tested, too?

Your blood passes through your kidneys, where it is purified and filtered; testing the urine can detect hormones and chemicals that have been purified from the blood and that may indicate serious conditions.[40] The urine is used basically as an index of the individual's health. By observing the color, weight, smell, acidity, and sediment in the urine, a doctor can detect early signs of serious disease.

The following elements present in the urine in too high a proportion can signal these disorders:

- *Protein*—kidney disease.

- *Sugar (glucose)*—diabetes.

- *Bilirubin*—obstruction of bile ducts or destruction of red blood cells.

- *Blood*—serious infection or disease of the kidneys or bladder, including cancer.

Some do-it-yourself medical tests are on the market today, including tests to measure occult blood in the stools, blood pressure, pregnancy, and sugar in the urine (a signal of diabetes). Though these tests can be valuable in supplementing medical testing as an early detection device, they should never be used to *replace* professional medical testing, especially because of the inaccuracy rates of some home do-it-yourself tests and the inabilities of people in accurately performing them.[41]

THE MEDICAL EXAMINATION

The blood and urine tests just described are part of what is considered to be a complete physical examination, although they may be ordered specially at other times you visit the doctor in order to help with diagnosis.

What else is routine as far as a physical examination goes? What should you expect as part of a complete physical?

A skilled doctor can examine you from head to toe, arrange for laboratory tests, ask questions, and uncover almost any existing disorder in a period of less than two hours by use of the complete physical examination. To begin with, the physician asks the patients questions—concerning complaints, sleeping habits, sexual habits, work habits, eating habits, family medical problems, medical history, drug use, significant injuries sustained in the past, allergies, exercise habits, and how much tea, coffee, alcohol, and tobacco the patient uses. With the answers to these questions the doctor already has a good preliminary picture of you by the time you enter the examining room for the actual physical.

The actual method varies among doctors, but a good physical examination should include a thorough check of the following:

THE EYES

In checking your eyes, the doctor will probably use an eye chart to test for visual acuity. She will then look at the external structures of the eyes such as the lids, the whites, and the membrane that covers the eye. In addition, she will undoubtedly test your pupil reaction to light. She may administer other tests such as having you follow her finger with your eyes or having you shift your focus from a close object to a distant one (this tests your eyes' ability to accommodate).

She will also want to observe the internal portions of the eye with an instrument called an ophthalmoscope. By using this instrument, she can note the appearance and normalcy of the vessels and other structures within the eye.

An examination such as this is helpful in the detection of diabetes, high blood pressure, or glaucoma.

THE EARS

Your doctor will begin his examination of the ears by looking at the outside of the ears and will then use an instrument called an otoscope (very similar in function to an ophthalmoscope) to look at the internal structures. He will also look for inflammation, infection, and blockages.

After looking at the internal and external ear, he will conduct some type of hearing test. It is common for a doctor to test hearing acuity by speaking softly and having you tell him what he has said. It is also a frequent practice to test the conductance of sound through air compared to the conductance through bone. To perform this test, the doctor will use a tuning fork.

THE NOSE, MOUTH, AND THROAT

For examination of the nose, your doctor will use the otoscope with different attachments. She will look at the lining of the nose for growths, bleeding, inflammation, and swelling. From the color and general appearance of the lining, she can diagnose various disease or allergy conditions.

The doctor will next examine your mouth. She will often use a penlight to illuminate the structures better. She will examine your cheeks, tongue, teeth, lips, gums, and roof of the mouth for any growths or other conditions that may signal disease.

THE NECK

As there are many glands in the neck area, the doctor will use his fingers to palpate this part of the body. He will generally palpate the salivary glands, the thyroid, and various lymph nodes for swelling or growths. Enlarged or tender glands or nodes may indicate infection elsewhere in the body.

THE LUNGS AND HEART

At this stage, the doctor will first observe the shape and symmetry of the chest. The general physical appearance of the chest can be a good indicator of disease. While looking at your chest, she will probably also note your breathing rate. Normal breathing rate is 16–20 breaths per minute.

The doctor may percuss or tap your chest and back with her fingers. The sounds she notes on percussion give a clue to the health of your lungs.

She will also listen to your lungs with a stethoscope. She will have you breathe deeply and listen to your breath sounds as you inhale and exhale.

After listening to the lungs, the doctor will use the stethoscope to listen to your heart. By noting heartbeat sounds, the doctor can become aware of abnormal conditions such as valve defects.

The doctor will also examine a woman's breasts. She will pay particular attention to the presence of lumps or other problems that may signal serious breast disease such as cancer.

THE ABDOMEN

By having you lie on your back, your doctor will note the outward appearance of your abdomen. He will look for signs of hernias, scars, pulsations, and masses. Next he will percuss, palpate, and use the stethoscope to determine as best he can the internal health of the abdominal organs. By listening to the abdomen through the stethoscope, he can determine the normalcy of bowel sounds. By pressing deeply with the hands, the doctor can feel the size and shape of the liver, spleen, stomach, and kidneys. Pain or tenderness may indicate abnormal conditions of these organs.

THE GENITALS

Women should receive an examination of the external genitals and a pelvic examination. In a pelvic exam, the doctor will use a speculum and gloved hand to check for infection or abnormalities of the cervix, vagina, uterus, fallopian tubes, and ovaries. A Pap test for the detection of cervical cancer is also part of the examination of a women's genitals.

In men, the examination will include observance of the external genitalia for abnormalities and palpation of the testicles for the presence of growths or tenderness. In addition, the physician will check the prostate during the rectal exam.

THE RECTUM

For performance of the rectal exam, the doctor will insert a lubricated and gloved finger into the anus. He will check for growths, tenderness, or other abnormalities.

If he believes that you may be at high risk for cancer, he may perform a sigmoidoscopy in which a lighted tube is passed into the colon so that he can examine its internal appearance. The doctor will palpate the male patient's prostate gland through the rectum for enlargement or other possible disease conditions.

THE ARMS, LEGS, AND FEET

The doctor will note movement of the extremities during the course of the examination, and she will also be aware of rashes, bruises, or other skin conditions that may not be normal. She will be especially aware of possible vein problems in the legs and will note any swelling that may occur in the ankles.

THE NERVOUS SYSTEM

The doctor will examine your reflexes, muscle strength, coordination, and stability as he performs the physical examination. Depending upon how well he knows you and your physical condition, he may perform a detailed or simple examination in this area.

DO YOU NEED AN ANNUAL CHECKUP?

Recent medical developments have caused doctors to question the need for an annual checkup of active, healthy people. You should certainly have an annual checkup (and sometimes a checkup at more frequent intervals) if you or your doctor determine that you are a member of a high-risk group and that you have a good possibility of developing some medical problem.

If you do not run the risk of developing specific medical problems, you probably don't need a complete physical checkup every year. There are some exceptions to this rule:[42]

If you have been exposed to tuberculosis or if you live in an area where tuberculosis is common, you should be tested every year for the disease. While chest X rays used to be the most common method of testing, you should ask for a tuberculin skin test instead in order to avoid unnecessary exposure to X ray.

If you are a female over the age of twenty-five, you should have a Pap smear every year. Women over twenty-five should also conduct breast self-examination each month and should have their breasts examined annually by a physician (this can be accomplished at the same time the Pap smear is taken).

After you reach the age of forty, you should be examined annually for glaucoma.

After you reach the age of thirty, you should have an annual examination that includes urine cultures, urinalysis, and tests for blood in the stools (to detect cancer of the digestive tract, kidneys, or bladder). After the age of fifty, you should have a sigmoidoscopy annually.

Your blood pressure should be checked at least once a year regardless of your sex or age.

MEDICAL INSURANCE

By the end of the last decade approximately 18 million Americans had no health insurance coverage; an additional 19 million Americans had health insurance that was inadequate or that did not cover hospital and physician charges. A total of 46 million Americans had health insurance that did not include coverage against large medical bills or catastrophic illnesses.[43]

You may be insured as a student through a policy that you paid for as part of your tuition, or you may be covered by a policy through your employer; some health insurance policies cover children up to a certain age, so you may still be covered on a parent's health or life insurance policy. But how can you determine if you have enough coverage?

Insurance policies are grouped into a number of categories that will help you determine generally what kind of coverage you have:[44]

- *Hospital expense policies,* which cover only the expenses of hospitalization (some policies cover only the cost of the hospital room and do not include laboratory costs or physician fees).
- *Hospital-surgical policies,* which cover some medical fees, the costs connected with surgery, and the cost of hospitalization.
- *Major-medical policies,* which pay for a broad range of medical, surgical, and hospital expenses.

- *Dread disease policies,* which pay expenses incurred only in connection with a specific disease (usually cancer, although "catastrophic illness" policies are available for coverage of some other diseases).

- *Accident policies,* which cover only those expenses incurred in connection with an accident.

- *Disability policies,* which pay a fixed income if you are unable to work due to an industrial accident, some other kind of accident, or illness. Disability policies do *not* pay for medical or hospital expenses; instead they pay you a fixed income, which you may spend as you desire.

Some insurance policies—labeled *selectively renewable*—can be dropped by the insurance companies for any of a number of reasons (other than a deterioration of the policyholder's health), and the premium payments can be increased by the health insurance company. Noncancelable and guaranteed-renewable policies are rarely sold today due to the explosive increase in medical expenses.

WHAT SHOULD YOUR INSURANCE POLICY INCLUDE?

To determine whether you are adequately covered by health insurance, check your policy. It should include the following as a standard of minimum coverage:[45]

Hospital insurance. For a maximum deductible fee of $100, you should have hospital expense coverage that includes hospital room and board, general nursing care, and special diets for at least twenty-one days of continuous confinement. Your hospital policy should cover at least 80 percent of a semiprivate room charge (in some areas, insurance pays a flat rate per day, such as $50; this may not come close to covering the costs considering the rapidly increasing hospitalization costs).

Your policy should also cover at least 80 percent of the costs for surgery, recovery room fees, equipment (such as wheelchairs), intensive care, drugs, vaccines, intravenous preparations, dressings, plaster casts, oxygen, anesthesia, physiotherapy, chemotherapy, X rays, electrocardiograms, radiation, or other customary hospital services rendered in connection with your hospitalization.

Your hospital policy should also cover outpatient services on the day surgery is performed or for a period of up to twenty-four hours following an accident. It also should cover at least 80 percent of the emergency room charges.

Medical insurance. Your policy should cover at least 80 percent of all surgical charges (including preoperative and postoperative care by a physician),

185

at least 80 percent of anesthetic charges, and at least 80 percent of all in-hospital medical services (including the physician's fee for a bed patient).

Major-medical insurance. Your policy should include maximum benefits of at least $10,000. You should have coverage (which ranges from policy to policy) for laboratory tests, X rays, drugs, radiation therapy, artificial limbs, treatment, and therapy performed outside a hospital.

If you are at risk of developing a critical disease and your risk is extremely high, you may want to consider taking out a catastrophic illness policy in addition to your regular health insurance (such a policy, for example, would cover expenses incurred from cancer). Since such policies are generally expensive, you should carefully evaluate your need for such a policy before enrolling for one.

PRESCRIPTION
AND OVER-THE-COUNTER DRUGS

In order to get the most out of the thousands of drugs that are available on the market today, you should know how to use those drugs effectively and which drugs to keep on hand. You should always have a few simple, safe, and effective medical supplies on hand at home. Periodically check your medicine chest and toss out any outdated prescriptions, unlabeled bottles, or medicines you no longer need (such as an ointment for a skin infection that has cleared up). To stock your medicine chest, get the following:[46]

Aspirin. Buy the least costly aspirin you can find. If you're allergic or sensitive to aspirin, buy a substitute that contains acetaminophen. If you don't use aspirin a great deal, buy the 100-tablet size bottle; if you have more frequent need for aspirin, buying it in large sizes can save you money. Check your aspirin from time to time to make sure it has not become crumbly (especially if you live in an area of high humidity). Keep your aspirin (and all other medical supplies) in a cool, dark place, and make sure all medications are capped tightly to prevent loss of potency or contamination.

Antacid. If you suffer only occasional indigestion or heartburn, sodium bicarbonate works well. Read the label of the medication carefully: Choose a simple antacid, not one that has been impregnated with medications for headache, constipation, insomnia, and so on. All the product should do is combat excess acidity.

Diarrhea remedy. A kaolin/pectin product is helpful in combatting diarrhea that stems from a mild intestinal infection or from tainted food. (If your diarrhea is more serious or if it lasts for a period longer than a few days, you should consult your physician for a prescription remedy.)

Antipruritic. You should have ordinary calamine lotion on hand for relief of skin irritation, rashes, insect bites, or poison ivy/oak contamination.

Antiseptic. The best antiseptic to have at home—and the only one generally needed—is isopropyl (70 percent) alcohol, usually purchased as rubbing alcohol.

Decongestant. Depending on the kind of medication you generally buy, you should have a small stock of decongestant on hand for those times when you are suddenly hit with a cold. (If you choose nasal sprays or nose drops, you should not purchase more than half an ounce at a time, since these tend to lose potency more quickly than decongestants in tablet or capsule form.)

Laxative. You should have a mild laxative—one containing methylcellulose, psyllium, or dioctyl sodium sulfosuccinate (read the label!)—on hand for occasional bouts with constipation. Dietary remedies (such as fruits or fruit juice) are best when combatting constipation.

First aid supplies. Your cache of first aid supplies will depend on the things you need most often, but, according to your needs, you may want to consider having on hand such items as adhesive tape, sterile gauze pads, tweezers, an ice bag, a heating pad or hot-water bottle, a clinical thermometer (oral or rectal), enema equipment (or a disposable enema), and Band-Aids.

THINGS YOU SHOULD NOT STOCK
You should not stock the following in your home medicine chest:

Antiseptics other than rubbing alcohol. These include iodine and mercury antiseptics (including mercurochrome or merthiolate).

Aromatic spirits of ammonia. Frequently recommended for fainting, these can be dangerous if used improperly.

Boric acid solutions or powders.

Cough syrups and elixirs. A cough lasting longer than a week should be checked by a physician; you should not attempt to mask the cough by using over-the-counter cough syrups or elixirs.

Over-the-counter burn ointments. Many of these contain chemicals that cause severe allergic reactions for many people. If a burn is too serious to be treated by cold running water, you should see a doctor.

REFERENCES

[1]Consumer's Union, *The Medicine Show,* revised and expanded (New York: Random House, Inc./Pantheon Books, Inc., 1976), p. 13.

[2] "Battle Begins over National Health Insurance," *U.S. News and World Report,* June 25, 1979, p. 62.

[3]*We Want You to Know About Television Radiation* (Rockville, Md.: U.S. Department of Health, Education and Welfare, Public Health Service), DHEW publication no. (FDA) 76-8041.

[4]Carl E. Willgoose, *Environmental Health* (Philadelphia: W. B. Saunders Company, 1979), p. 1.

[5]Roger S. Mitchell, Franklyn N. Judson, Thomas S. Moulding, Phillip Weiser, Loring J. Brock, David L. Kelble, and Joseph Pollard, "Health Effects of Urban Air Pollution," *JAMA,* 242, no. 11 (September 14, 1979), 1163.

[6]This and the information on effects and costs of air pollution adapted from Brent Q. Hafen, ed., *Man, Health, and Environment* (Minneapolis: Burgess Publishing Co., 1972), pp. 42–70.

[7] "Winners and Losers," from "Special Report: Water," *Family Health,* 6 (September), p. 33.

[8] "Home Water Filters: Cancer Fighters or Money Wasters?" from "Special Report: Water," p. 42.

[9]Kenneth L. Jones, Louis W. Shainberg, and Curtis O. Beyer, *Environmental Health* (San Francisco: Canfield Press, 1971), p. 8.

[10]Gladwin Hill, *Cleansing Our Waters* (New York: Public Affairs Committee, 1974), p. 3.

[11]Environmental Protection Agency, *Clean Water and the Dairy Products Industry* (Washington, D.C.: U.S. Government Printing Office, July 1976), p. 2.

[12]Ibid., p. 8.

[13]Environmental Protection Agency, *Hazardous Wastes* (Washington, D.C.: U.S. Government Printing Office, 1975), p. 13.

[14]Ibid.

[15]Hill, *Cleansing Our Waters,* p. 2.

[16]Ibid.

[17]Ibid.

[18]Ibid.

[19]"How Unseen Microwaves Are Changing Your Life," *U.S. News and World Report,* December 9, 1974, p. 31.

[20]*We Want You to Know About Microwave Oven Radiation* (Rockville, Md.: U.S. Department of Health, Education and Welfare, Public Health Service), DHEW publication no. (FDA) 73-8049, pp. 2–4.

[21]Roger R. Shipley and Carolyn G. Plonsky, *Consumer Health* (New York: Harper & Row, 1980), pp. 138–39.

[22]Lewis Miller, *The Life You Save* (New York: William Morrow & Co., Inc., 1979), p. 28.

[23]From *The Whole Health Catalogue* by Shirley Linde, p. 4. Copyright © 1977 by Shirley Linde. Reprinted with permission of Rawson, Wade.

[24]Adapted from pp. 85–91 in *The Life You Save* by Lewis Miller. Copyright © 1979 by Lewis Miller. By permission of William Morrow & Company.

[25]Adapted from Miller, *The Life You Save,* pp. 94–98. Copyright © 1979 by Lewis Miller. By permission of William Morrow & Company.

[26]Linde, *Whole Health Catalogue,* pp. 6–7. Copyright © 1977 by Shirley Linde. Reprinted with permission of Rawson, Wade.

[27]Ibid., pp. 7–8.

[28]"Inside Our Hospitals," *U.S. News and World Report,* March 5, 1979, pp. 34–35.

[29]Adapted from Miller, *The Life You Save,* pp. 164–70. Copyright © 1979 by Lewis Miller. By permission of William Morrow & Company.

[30]Adapted from Miller, *The Life You Save,* pp. 171–78. Copyright © 1979 by Lewis Miller. By permission of William Morrow & Company.

[31]Linde, *Whole Health Catalogue,* pp. 132–34. Copyright © 1977 by Shirley Linde. Reprinted with permission of Rawson, Wade.

[32]Aaron E. Klein, *Medical Tests and You* (New York: Grosset & Dunlap, Inc., 1977), p. 13.

[33]Ibid., pp. 8–9.

[34]"X Ray Hazards—Real and Imagined," *Science Digest,* March 1979, p. 82.

[35]The New Worry over X Rays and What You Can Do Aobut It," *Good Housekeeping,* July 1979, p. 221.

[36]Ibid.

[37]"Growing Debate over Dangers of Radiation," *U.S. News and World Report,* May 14, 1979, p. 26; *We Want You to Know About Diagnostic X-Rays* (Rockville, Md.: U.S. Department of Health, Education and Welfare, Public Health Service), DHEW publication no. (FDA) 73-8048.

[38]*Did You as a Child or a Young Adult Have X-ray Treatments Involving Your Head or Neck?* (Rockville, Md.: U.S. Department of Health, Education and Welfare, Public Health Service, National Institutes of Health), DHEW publication no. (NIH) 77-1206, pp. 1–3.

[39]Genell Subak-Sharpe, "The Tests That Tell (Nearly) All," *Family Health,* September, p. 41.

[40]Ibid., p. 42.

[41]"Medical Tests You Do on Yourself," *Changing Times,* August 1979, pp. 13–15.

[42]Donald M. Vickery and James F. Fries, *Take Care of Yourself: A Consumer's Guide to Medical Care* (Reading, Mass.: Addison-Wesley Publishing Co., Inc., 1976), p. 12.

[43]"Battle Begins over National Health Insurance," p. 62.

[44]"How to Shop for Health Insurance," (Washington, D.C.: U.S. Department of Health, Education, & Welfare, 1978), DHEW publication 78-619, pp. 2–5.

[45]Ibid., p. 8.

[46]*Medicine Chest,* pp. 306–13.

INDEX

Aspirin, 107, 123–24, 152, 174, 185–86
Asthma, 116–19, 155–56, 182
Atherosclerosis, 45, 47, 49, 53, 55–58
Atria, 42
Automobile exhaust, 75, 153–54

BARIUM ENEMA, 85
Basal cell cancers, 86–87
Bee sting allergy, 117, 121
Belladonna, 124
Bicarbonates, 159
Bile ducts, obstruction of, 179–80
Bilirubin, 179–80
Biofeedback, 29
Biopsies, 85, 106
Birth control (*see* Condom; Contraceptives; Oral contraceptives)
Blacks:
  and breast cancer, 79
  and high blood pressure, 8, 46
  and sickle-cell anemia, 8
  and skin cancer, 87
Blood:
  circulation, 4, 42–43, 115
  clots, 49–50, 54, 56–57
  donation of, 175
  pressure, 4, 45–49, 108, 121, 165, 167–68, 180, 182–83
  in stools, 84, 124, 180, 183
  tests, 43, 114–15, 165, 178–80, 183
  transmission of cancer cells through, 70–71
Blue babies, 60
Blurred vision, 157
Boredom, 6, 31
Boric acid solutions, 187
Botulism, 132
Bowel habits, 84–85, 169
Breast:
  cancer, 77–80, 182; linked to guilt/depression, 27; linked to hormones, 73, 80, 84; linked to oral contraceptives, 76, 80; linked to stress, 83; risk factors in developing, 79, 82–84, 89; surgery for, 78–79, 82–83; victims, death rate among, 77
  change in contour of, 81, 97
  exam by doctor, 80, 164, 182
  large masses in, 82, 97
  lumps in, 77–82, 89, 97, 182
  self-examination of, 6, 80–82, 97, 100, 183
  tumors, 69, 77–82
  variety in texture of, 80

Bronchial asthma, 117, 153, 155–56
Bronchial tubules, 155
Bronchioles, 155–56
Bronchitis, 93, 153, 156, 182
Bursa, 110
Bursitis, 110

CALCIFICATION:
  detected by fluoroscope, 44
Calcium, 158, 179
Calomine lotion, 186
Cancer, 67–103
  age factor in developing, 79–80, 83, 89–90
  causes of, 72–76
  diagnosing, 95
  environmental causes of, 72, 74–77
  heredity a factor in developing, 7, 72, 79, 83, 89–91, 167
  incidence of, 76–77
  nature of, 68–72
  personality-type prone to, 27, 73
  preventing, 99–101
  risk factors in developing, 91–95
  specific kinds of, 77–90
  stress a cause of, 8, 27
  surgical treatment for, 85, 97–98
  treatments, 97–99
  victims, death rate among, 4, 8, 67, 76–77, 84, 86
  X rays used to treat, 177
Capillaries, 42–43
Carbohydrates, 53, 111, 179
Carbon:
  dioxide, 42–43
  monoxide, 153, 157
Cardiac:
  arrest due to insect sting, 121
  catheter, 45
  rhythms, 24
Carotid arteriogram, 176
Carter, President Jimmy, 3
Catastrophic illness, 161, 183, 185
Central nervous system, 158
Cervix, cancer of, 27, 90, 148, 182
Chemicals, carcinogenic, 74–75, 93
Chemotherapy, 85, 97–98
Chest X rays, 177
Chickenpox (Varicella), 132
Childbirth, 162
Chloride, 159
Chlorine, 75, 157

194